Your Heart Beats for Him

A Caregiver's Heart Transplant Journey

Pamela Wareham Washnock

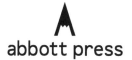
abbott press

Abbott Press books may be ordered through booksellers or by contacting:

Abbott Press
1663 Liberty Drive
Bloomington, IN 47403
www.abbottpress.com
Phone: 1 (866) 697-5310

ISBN: 978-1-4582-2126-1 (sc)
ISBN: 978-1-4582-2127-8 (e)

Library of Congress Control Number: 2017912745

Print information available on the last page.

Abbott Press rev. date: 08/31/2017

Contents

Acknowledgements vii
Dedication ix
Your Heart Beats For Him xi
Preface.. xiii

Chapter 1:   How It All Began.. 1
Chapter 2:   Life Leading Up To Transplant 3
Chapter 3:   LVAD Surgery..7
Chapter 4:   Waiting For A Donor Heart 97
Chapter 5:   The New Heart 107
Chapter 6:   Going Home 126
Chapter 7:   Back To Work 144

Epilogue: One Year and Beyond Post Transplant........ 147
Death Was Not An Option 149
Medications.. 161

Acknowledgements

We would like to thank my good friend Candy Bravo for her time and effort in helping me write this book, which started out as only notes from a journal I kept while Bob was going through this journey.

Also, a big thank you, which doesn't seem quite enough, to the Doctors, Nurses, and Staff of the Mayo Hospital Heart Transplant Team and ICU Team in Phoenix, Arizona, for their excellent care and kindness. Without them, Bob would not be here today.

Thank you to David Kazalski who created the cover, which is the art genre called "Steam Punk."

I would also like to thank all our family and friends, for their prayers, cards, gifts and flowers.

Last but not least, I need to Thank God. I guess He just wasn't through with Bob yet; He has more for him to do in this lifetime.

Dedication

This story would not have a happy ending if it were not for the selfless, generous, heart-wrenching decision by a family to allow their loved one's heart to be donated when life was no longer a viable option.

We don't know who you are, but if not for you, I would not have my husband, our children and grandchildren would not have their father and grandfather, and our friends would have lost a wonderful man.

Please accept my sincere undying gratitude, and may you find some comfort in knowing that this heart is strong and so dearly accepted to prolong life and happiness.

Thank you

Your Heart Beats For Him

My name is Pam. I want to share my story with others who might be facing what my husband Bob and I have been living with for the past several years - the ups and downs of declining health, to the need for a heart transplant, and through the process of transplant and life beyond. My hope is that if I can help one other person to understand what it was like, and to know there is hope and light at the end of a very long tunnel, then my effort will be worth it. You must understand that our experience may be different from others.

There are several books written from the standpoint of the heart transplant patient. My book is dedicated to the spouses of the patients, and the Care Givers, because you have a difficult journey ahead of you, too.

Preface

Bob and I met in college at Michigan Tech University; he was a member of a fraternity and we had three fun years of college together. I first noticed Bob in golf class, and then later met him through mutual friends. During his last year of college I moved to Lower Peninsula of Michigan, but we still dated through his graduation. My mother threw Bob a graduation party, which his mother and sister attended. We really had a great relationship, or so I thought.

After graduation, Bob took a job in Utah, and we drifted apart and had other relationships. Bob had two children from his marriage, and I remained single. We rediscovered each other during the fall of 1981, when Bob located me through mutual friends, got my phone number, and eventually called me. The rest is history - a love story for real. Bob and I were married in June of 1983.

CHAPTER 1

How It All Began

Bob was a vibrant, active man during his years leading up to this story. He was a hockey referee for high school and pee-wee leagues, an avid snow and water skier, rode motorcycles, drove a Corvette, light drinker, non-smoker except for an occasional cigar. He was a healthy man.

Bob went skiing with a friend in Colorado one winter day in 1997, and started having a hard time catching his breath. He thought it was altitude sickness. Cutting his skiing trip short, he returned to Tucson where we lived at that time, and his condition did not improve. We decided to visit his doctor, who asked many questions such as his travel history, family history, and exposure to any virus or other sicknesses. Initial diagnosis was "heart problems," but we couldn't figure out what was causing it; we later discovered there was heart disease on his mother's side of the family.

Under a cardiologist's care, we began our long journey.

1

Bob was given medications for a few years, which helped his heart function. But in 2000, the doctors detected abnormal heart rhythms and said that if his heart were to start beating too fast he could pass out and not wake up; in other words, it could be fatal. So an ICD device was implanted, which would detect abnormal rhythms and shock the heart back to a normal rhythm. He lived with this device for many years, and had to give up motorcycle riding, because if he were to get shocked while on his bike, it could be fatal. When he would get shocked, it was like a mule kicking him in the chest; he was once shocked while sitting on a bar stool and it knocked him off the stool. Needless to say, motorcycle riding was no longer an activity he could do safely, so he sold his bike and bought a 2002 yellow Corvette convertible. Pretty good trade, as far as I was concerned.

Over the years, Bob was airlifted from small towns we lived in to larger cities with better health care. Several times he had oblations, a procedure where an electrode is inserted into your heart from a peripheral artery. Then the doctor carefully burns areas in the heart that cause arrhythmias. Medications and oblations wouldn't strengthen his heart, but could lengthen the time before needing a transplant.

CHAPTER 2

Life Leading Up To Transplant

Finally in 2009, Bob's EP (Cardiac Electrophysiologist-the science of elucidating, diagnosing and treating the electrical activities of the heart) recommended he contact the Mayo Clinic in Phoenix, Arizona, for an evaluation for a heart transplant. After talking with the transplant team, it was determined that Bob was still "too healthy" at this point, but at least he was on the books, so to speak, and they were familiar with him if and when the time should come.

We were living about five hours from Phoenix and would make several trips to doctors over a two-year period. Then the company Bob was working for transferred him closer to Phoenix, and we bought a home in Sun City Grand located in Surprise, Arizona. Bob worked at a mine about 1 ½ hours away, and he would commute to the mine during the week and then be at our home in Surprise on the weekends.

A couple more years passed, working, traveling, and living life. In August of 2011, Bob was starting to become more tired, shortness of breath was getting worse, and he was having a hard time walking just a matter of feet. He would come home for lunch and then take a nap to get him through the rest of the day.

In September of 2011, we returned to the Mayo Clinic, and it was determined that he would need a new heart, so he began the process of testing, questions, and evaluations to determine if he was a good candidate for a transplant. During this time Bob continued to work full time. We really didn't realize the extent or severity of his situation at this time, although he was always so very tired.

We had planned a trip to Las Vegas for the end of October to see "America's Got Talent" show, thinking that if he couldn't walk we would use a wheelchair to get him around, but at an office visit just the day before we were to leave the doctor said, "NO, I do not recommend you go to Las Vegas, and you're lucky I don't put you in the hospital right now." He also informed Bob that he was not to return to work, but go home for the weekend and, "We will see you on Monday."

Wow, were we in shock, scared - what were we going to do? We knew he couldn't live this way, and something had to be done. We talked about going on disability, but Bob said he could use his vacation time for now. So we didn't make any decisions about his job or disability at this time.

When we returned on Monday, they admitted Bob

to the hospital because his heart function was extremely low. I believe he had a 7-10% ejection fraction, a number that determines how well the heart is pumping, with a normal person having maybe 50-75%. He was given a PICC Line (peripherally inserted central catheter), which delivers medication closer to the heart in his case. This was to help his heart function, and it seemed to be helping.

While in the hospital, Bob finished the evaluation for a Transplant, and was approved and listed on the Transplant List on November 9th, 2011, as a 2-B status, not the highest on the list, because his heart was being helped by the IV medication. The highest status on the list is a 1-A. He remained in the hospital for a couple of weeks, so I would go home every night, a forty-five minute drive each way, and return in the morning.

In the middle of his hospital stay, our home at the mine site needed to be cleaned out. Bob was in the hospital under great care so this was a good time for me to pack up our home; it took me a couple of days with help from friends. We packed the home, sold most of our furniture, and hired a moving company to move our belongings to a storage unit close to our home in Surprise. Since we couldn't afford to take care of two homes not knowing when Bob would be going back to work, this had to be done.

When he was released from the hospital, we went home with an IV Pump, that I had learned how to change and flush out the lines, and also how to change the IV bag. Home Health Care came by daily to check on Bob - take his vitals, blood pressure, temperature, check his PICC Line, and to change the dressing every three days. This continued, going to the doctor and changing the IV medications, for about seven weeks, until Christmas of 2011. Just before Christmas they really wanted to admit Bob to the hospital, but said they would wait a few days.

December 25, 2011, was not a happy day, as Bob slept most of the day. He did manage to open gifts, but he did not feel like eating since he had no appetite, due to his poor heart function. Looking back, he probably should have been in the hospital, but after all, it was Christmas, and Bob loved Christmas time. I received a tablet as a gift, but I really wasn't sure if I wanted one or not. Little did I know how it would help keep me sane over the next weeks and months to come!

CHAPTER 3

LVAD Surgery

On December 26th, we woke up and Bob was not feeling well at all, so we called the Clinic and off we went to the Emergency Room. The IV medication he was on was not working as well as planned, so he was admitted to the hospital, and we were informed they wanted to insert a Heart Pump to help his heart while he was waiting for a new heart. We were all hoping that a donor heart would come over the next week so that we didn't need to insert the pump, but it didn't.

Bob had the pump inserted, and after surgery was in ICU recovering. He was now moved up on the Transplant List to a 1-A, the highest you can be on the list, since he was now in critical condition. This was such a trying time for me, waiting to see what would happen, praying that a donor heart would become available, but yet again knowing someone had to lose a loved one in order for Bob to live.

If a heart did not come in the next few days, we were educated on implanting another device called an LVAD (Left Ventricular Assist Device). This device would help his heart to pump more blood throughout the body to save the other organs. The worry here was that his organs were not getting enough blood flow and they would start to deteriorate.

I am so grateful that we now lived close enough for me to go home every night. I believe a Higher Being was watching over us, for Bob to be transferred to a larger city where he could have easy access to excellent medical care.

I would arrive first thing in the morning carrying my overnight bag, because I never knew when a heart would come, and I would want to stay close to the hospital if one did. I lived with my cell phone by my side and an overnight bag in the car, just waiting for the call. But no call came.

It was now January 2nd, 2012, and the doctors informed us that they couldn't wait any longer for a donor heart and would have to do the surgery to implant the LVAD. We agreed that this is the best way to keep Bob's organs working while waiting for a donor heart. Bob and I had our talk about what to do if he did not make it through the surgery; we cried and hugged. We were both so scared, but this was the only way to save his life. He would die without this surgery; his heart is just too weak. Surgery was scheduled for January 4th and I decided to stay in a hotel so that I could be nearby and not have to drive home and back again while waiting for him to get out of surgery.

The surgery was first thing in the morning on January 4th. We were able to see each other before he went into surgery, and we said our "see-you- laters," because good-bye just didn't seem right. At this point he was taken off the Transplant List until he recovered from the LVAD surgery.

When he was taken into surgery, one of the nurses gave me a brochure that said what to do when you have a loved one in the hospital. It stated to take care of yourself, because your loved one will need you when they start to recover, and also to journal your days to help remember what has happened, because when you are under this much stress you really can't remember all the details. (I started to journal my thoughts and what was happening to Bob with medication, surgery, etc. This became a journal of the days and weeks of tedium and frustration, of pain and discomfort. It's not a fun or a happy story. A lot of the journaling was clinical, like medications, machines, when he was given what, but also what I did and my feelings while he was in the hospital.)

I went back to the hotel to wait; I was told they would call me when the surgery was over and I could see him. Those four hours seemed to take forever. The doctors called me and said the surgery went well, but because of Bob's heart functions and retention of fluids, his body was dilated, and they couldn't close the incision, so they just covered the incision with surgical gauze and something like a big band aid. I could see him soon; he would be brought back to ICU.

I went back to the hospital to wait and when I was able to see him, they told me he would be sedated until they could close the incision. At this point I was so tired, Bob was sedated, and so I just sat, waiting, worrying and crying; it was so hard to see him just lying there, connected to machines. I stayed another night at the hotel then went back to the hospital early the next morning, although I couldn't get in to see him until 9:00 a.m.

January 5th. Bob was still completely sedated. They took out the balloon pump from his groin, since the LVAD was functioning as it should. He will be sedated for a few days until he can be closed from surgery. I am told to go home, rest, and that I will be called if anything happens; I can call anytime I want to check on his status. Bob was stable at this point, although I felt so guilty to leave, but yet what could I do, just sit and look at him? I called my sister and asked her what she thought. She thought it would be a good idea to go home, as long as the hospital staff thinks it okay. So I said my goodnight to Bob, and drove home. So restless, I couldn't sit still.

I began to take down our Christmas tree and decorations, crying most of the time because Bob wouldn't see this year's Christmas again, and of course I was so worried. I called the nurse on duty for Bob and was told that he was resting comfortably, and they would call if there were any changes. I did get a good night's sleep, because it seemed I hadn't had any rest for days.

January 6th, Friday. I arrived by 9:00 a.m., and the nurse filled me in on his night. Bob developed a temperature, therefore the blood vessels expanded, so when they tried to close him up again the heart didn't like it, meaning his blood pressure went up and the numbers on his LVAD weren't right. So they washed him out and a new dressing was applied.

A couple more days passed to see if they could close. It was such a trying time of waiting, Bob sedated in ICU, which is extremely intense, and I just wait and wonder what is next. Nurses said he was doing well.

During the night a nurse tried to wake him a little, and he did follow commands such as to squeeze her hand. I thought, "He is in there somewhere." He was connected to so many different IVs, I think I counted nine, he was on a ventilator because he couldn't breathe on his own, nitric oxide machine (it's a gas that helps the lungs function), drainage tubes, air bags for circulation in his legs, then there was the LVAD machine itself at the end of the bed, which gives readings as to how the LVAD is performing.

Get Well Cards and balloons from friends had started to arrive, and although he can't have flowers in ICU, some arrive at home. I took pictures of them so he can at least see them.

The brochure also advised starting an email of his progress. I started to send family and friends updates, and then they sent them on to others that may be interested, such as his professional groups. My sister sent them to my family and his brother sent them on to Bob's family. It helped keep everyone informed, and took some pressure off me. It was a great idea, and I did receive emails from family and friends and would read them to him while he was "sleeping." I was told he could hear me even though he doesn't respond.

The next few days, January 8-10th, 2012, his temperature was up and down, lots of lab work being done daily; lab results looked good, with liver and kidneys responding to the increase of blood flow. He is also started on nutrition through a GI tube/feeding tube going into the stomach. Surgery to close was cancelled again, as his temperature was still a little high and it needed to be normal for at least twenty-four hours before they try again; it's just not the right time. More testing; ECHO to see how the right heart is doing; results came back the same, which was good - at least the heart was not getting worse. The doctors were in as they were every day, but they all agreed it's going to be a long process. Lots of cultures were taken to see if there was an infection since his temperature was high, and it will take a few days to get the results.

Today Bob's sister Janice told his Mom that he had a pump inserted to help his heart. We think she understood, but Mom has dementia, and has a hard time seeing and hearing.

Nurses were keeping him very comfortable; washed his hair and a bath today, and he looked so nice. My friend Judy and I went to lunch. This was always a good break for me during the day. She is such a good friend, and she understands since her husband had a heart condition as well, but was not of good health otherwise for a transplant, and had passed away.

It was another long day in ICU. I said my goodnight, kissed and hugged Bob and said, "I love you." Went home and tried to sleep. Had a rough night; woke at 3:30 a.m. worried about the cultures they took. We were waiting to make sure he did not have any infections, which would not be good. If the LVAD were to get infected it would get into his blood and this could be fatal, so they were watching and concerned about temperatures as well.

These last few days were just more of the same, waiting. Sometimes I just don't know how I got through them.

Prayers and good wishes from family and friends, knowing he will wake up eventually, all these things helped.

January 11th. When I arrived, Bob had been to the operating room and was finally closed up, after a week of waiting. Doctor said that it went well, and he was responding well; numbers looked good. Doctors were watching him really closely and he was holding steady, which made them happy, and when the doctors are happy I felt things may be looking up. It was a long week of waiting and now ready for recovery.

Bob was being weaned off sedation drugs slowly, because if not he could have had withdrawals. More cultures taken today, tests, and temperature is up and down. It really was a good day getting the incision closed. When I got home there were a couple of messages from friends, but when I went to retrieve them and heard Bob's recorded voice on the machine, I broke down and cried, because it was the first time I had heard his voice in days. What a great sound.

January 12-14th. The weaning off drugs continued; also had what is called a "mini vacation" from the drugs last night for about 45 minutes to see if he would respond, and he did. Also taken off NO2 nitric oxide, but still on the ventilator.

Our favorite nurse had been with Bob through most of the time here in ICU and she needed some time off; today was her last day for a while. She has been wonderful, such an angel; she really wants to hear Bob's voice and meet him.

The evening nurse shaved, bathed, and washed his hair. Daily he was waking up a little more but still very sleepy; he was obeying commands like squeezing hands, although still on a ventilator. My days were sitting by Bob's side, talking to him, journaling, sending emails, passing time playing games on my tablet. I was told he can hear me, so I talked a lot, telling him that the neighbors stop me in the mornings and ask how he's doing, how everyone is concerned, how I went to a caregivers meeting which was helpful to know I am not alone and others are going through the same thing I am.

The Mayo Clinic had a celebration for 100 Heart Transplants in the lobby; it was a nice event with a lot of the former Heart Transplant patients there, doing so well.

Bob's sedation drugs have been stopped; he was opening his eyes a little more. They took out the Swan Line today; this is the line that measures pressures and other criteria. A rectal tube was inserted to help clean him out since he has been in bed for over two weeks now and has not eliminated; he cleaned out real good, will leave it at that. Working on getting him off the ventilator, but still not strong enough or awake enough. We watched a hockey game tonight; first time he seemed interested in anything, but he didn't seem to remember. It's okay; at least I could see his eyes open, although he couldn't talk because of the breathing tube.

January 15th. Bob has been in ICU, in bed, since December 26th. He is so weak and losing muscle; it's hard for him to lift his head, although he really tries. Physical Therapy came in for the first time to help with range of motion in bed, since he has been motionless for weeks, and he needs to start moving. Respiratory is working on getting him off the ventilator - there are some tests that are done to determine if he is strong enough and awake enough, and success comes at 2:15 p.m. - his breathing tube comes out.

We are so happy, I cry, I laugh, and the nurses are happy as well. I said to one nurse, "I wonder what his first words will be," she said, "Water," and lo and behold his first word was "Water." He can't have much, but he wants the pink spongy thing with water to suck on; he is limited because he may swallow the wrong way and get water into the lungs. They are very careful on how much he can have.

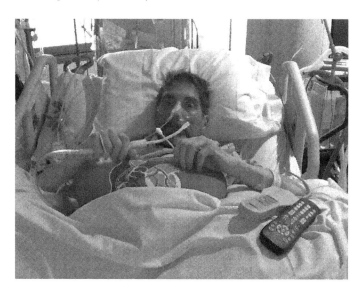

Bob in ICU after his LVAD surgery

Bob's breathing was very fast because he is weak and is having trouble breathing on his own, so at 5:15 p.m. he went back on the Ventilator. I'm so sad, began crying, wondering when will this all end, it's such a nightmare. I have to leave the room while they sedate him and put the breathing tube back in. It was such a happy day and then again so sad - what a roller coaster ride, and I don't *like* roller coasters. He is asleep again. It was such a joyous couple of hours, when he could talk to me a little. Now we wait again. They want to keep him quiet for a day or so. I go home to rest and I will see him tomorrow.

When I arrive on the 16th, his legs were being wrapped with an ace bandage to help with the swelling caused from fluid retention. Resting again today, a little awake, but not awake enough for the breathing tube to come out; maybe tomorrow they can remove it. An uneventful day, but a stressful one nonetheless, seeing him lie there wanting water he can't have, trying to talk and can't, trying to write on an eraser board, but too weak to hold a pen. I said my good night, a kiss and "I love you." Went home a little early tonight to do laundry; life does go on and these things have to get done.

The next day Physical Therapy was in moving his legs, and they tried to get him to sit up for the first time since Dec.26th. They got him sitting up with lots of help and really they had to hold him in a seated position or he would have fallen over onto the bed.

He is much more awake today, but very agitated about the ventilator, plus he is thirsty and can't have anything. Frustrated, he wants to talk but can't. He motioned that he is pissed off. It may sound funny, but this was his best day in three weeks. I had lunch with Judy while Bob napped. A long day, but a good one; he was stronger this afternoon. Wished Bob a good night's sleep before I left. Off I go home to rest, have a glass of wine, and sleep. Praying for another good day tomorrow.

January 18th. What a great day!!! My prayers have been answered. I had stopped for gas on my way to the hospital and my phone rang; it was the hospital. Immediately my heart sank, but it was his nurse, telling me Bob came off the ventilator at 8:15 a.m. and he is asking for me. This was the first time he was able to talk to me in two weeks. I told him that I was on my way and would be there in a few minutes. I was so excited and called my sister to say, "Bob just talked to me." I was crying but I knew I had to drive and keep calm. It was truly an exciting morning. He told me, "I am flying on my way to recovery now." He hasn't lost his sense of humor. So good to see and talk to him.

I filled him in on some of what had been happening; he doesn't remember most of it because of the drugs he has been on. Physical Therapy sat him on the edge of the bed and he actually stood for a couple of minutes, they had him do a few other exercises. Slow and steady he goes. All Bob wants is water, he is so thirsty, but has to wait until they can do a swallow test to make sure his throat muscles are working properly.

He is asking me questions like, "What happened when I fell out of the boat; are they selling the hospital?" Why? I don't know, still loopy from the drugs I guess. It is 2:30 p.m. and he wants to go home, and at 3:30 the ventilator went out the door, yeah, we are happy, no more ventilator. He asked for chocolate and water but I have to say NO. He asked me why am I so hard to get along with, so I gave him a pink spongy and said, "See, I am not so hard to get along with after all," and he said "No, you're just a pain in the ass." We laughed. At 3:30 he started to call his pink sponge a "wee nip." This is what a friend of ours used to call a cocktail. We laughed - so good to laugh for a change instead of crying all the time. Bob continues to ask how much the pink swabs cost, just confused. Then out of the blue he said, "I'm dying here, I am so thirsty, this is ridiculous." I said, "This isn't the Ritz," and he said, "Pretty damn close." And we laughed again. He seems awake but still under the influence.

Before I left for the day he told me to "Bring me an eff-in canteen tomorrow, you know the kind the cowboys wear on their saddles. I want water!!!" And we laughed again. I only (happy) cried once today, when I found out he came off the ventilator. Said goodnight and home I go for a good night's sleep. We had such a good day.

January 19th. Another sad day. The phone rang at 6:00 a.m., and my heart skipped a beat or two. It was the ICU doctor, telling me that they had to put Bob back on the ventilator because he was having trouble breathing and needed help; he is just too weak, she told me. So much progress was made yesterday, and here we are again. I just sat and bawled. After a little while I composed myself and went for a walk to clear my head. I usually try to get my walk in most mornings, since I sit around the rest of the day, also it's taking care of myself and that's what I am told to do. It's such a roller coaster ride.

I told him when I arrived, "You made it 20 hours off the vent, and the next time it will be for good. We have so many people praying for you, God will see us through." My sister's friend said, "God has a plan, we don't know what it is, but we must have faith he will bring us through this."

Bob's ECHO for the right side of the heart showed improvement today, and that is because of the LVAD doing its job. Doctors were surprised to see him back on the vent when they did their rounds this morning, and said, "We know you can do it, just get stronger." Everyone is praying for you, to get your strength.

There was talk today about putting in a tracheostomy to help his breathing but his surgeon said to wait, get some of this fluid off, and see what tomorrow brings. The tracheostomy would just be another place for an infection to possibly start, and we don't need that.

Our social worker was in and wrote on your Heart Pillow; it's given to heart patients so they have something to squeeze when they cough, and usually people write nice things on it. Awake all day, no naps, finally fell asleep around 5 p.m. and was still sleeping at 7:00, so I left to go home. I was watching the hockey game on TV and the Red Wings and Coyotes were playing in overtime in a shootout. The last Red Wing was going in for a goal and I said, "Goal for Bobbie, goal for Bobbie!" and he scored, Wings win.

I called to see how Bob was doing before I went to bed as I do every night, and he was still sleeping; I guess he got pooped out today. I pray that he sleeps all night. A few cards from friends came today; so nice to know so many people are thinking of him.

I cry a lot, to and from the hospital, I cry myself to sleep, and I wonder WHY?? I cry so much, then tonight it dawned on me that I cry because I AM SCARED, yes scared, of what is going to happen next, of the unknown. Bob has been in ICU twenty-six days now, and no sign of getting out anytime soon.

19

January 20th, Friday. The surgeon and the ICU doctors were in to see Bob for about half an hour, figuring out a plan for today. Still more fluids have to come off, and sleep as much as possible so he can get stronger to handle coming off the vent, maybe in the next twenty-four hours they will try again. I brought his Red Wings hat; he gave me a thumbs-up and was happy to have a hat. Everyone said how Bob looks good in his hat. A half hour of physical therapy today, but very hard to do with all the tubes attached to his body. A really quiet day, just what we needed. I left a little early and went to Happy Hour with Judy and then home, although I called to see how Bob was doing before I went to bed; he was still sleeping, so he didn't miss me.

January 21-22. When I arrived this morning, what a wonderful surprise I found – Bob was sitting in a chair (his bed converted to a chair position) and off the vent. He wanted to surprise me and he did! He was taken off the vent at 6 a.m. and sat in a chair from 8:00-10:30.

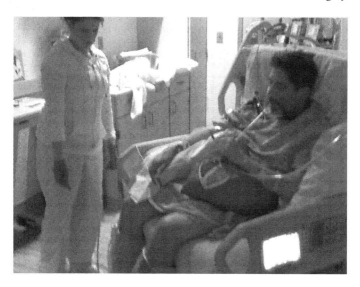

Bob with Nurse Sitting Up for the 1st Time

I got Bob cleaned up today, shaved, washed and fixed his hair. Looking good. Today just a little activity, since the last time he came off the vent I think he tried to do too much and got pooped out and had to go back on the vent the next day. Talking a lot today, telling me stories. One story was, "We were in an airplane and there were terrorists, a horn would sound and a seat would fall out of the plane through the floor into the Great Salt Lake." You also said that one of your doctors was on the plane, and I was one of the people that fell out of the plane into the lake; that's why you asked me why I wasn't wet, because the Coast Guard must have picked me up. Crazy dreams and talk because of the meds.

Still very thirsty, but have to wait until Monday, when a swallow test will be done, before he can have anything to swallow. For now just the pink swabs. Thirty minutes of Physical Therapy today, and napped for a couple of hours. I tried to nap as well, but no luck, so I just played on my tablet, and kept notes. Went for dinner and when I got back, Bob said I looked tired and that I should go home, so I left at 6:45 p.m., while he was watching hockey. But I called as usual to say goodnight.

The next day was a little busy for a Sunday. Drainage tubes came out around 5:00 p.m., plus Physical Therapy, and sitting in your chair. Watched football. The doctors said you are looking stronger and you can lift your arms so much better. One of the nurses came in and said that Bob would have one of two nurses next, but he didn't know which one. After he left I said, "Now the nurses are fighting over you," and he said, "I am one good looking son of a gun, why wouldn't they?" We laughed.

January 23rd, Monday. One month today since Bob was admitted into the hospital, twenty-nine of those days in ICU. Wow, it's been a long road and we have a long way to go. Patience please, dear God, and thank you for getting us this far.

A preliminary swallow test - he will swallow a dye, and a picture will be taken of his throat to make sure he can swallow, since he was on the ventilator for so long. He passed the swallow test with flying colors, so this means he can now start on liquids and maybe get the feeding tube out of his nose tomorrow.

Bob said, "Physical Therapy has been working my ass off this morning." It's 10:30 a.m. and Bob is very ornery. He is upset because he doesn't want another PICC Line put in today, but there is protocol for the amount of time these lines can stay in before they are changed out, and the time limit is up for this one. He is very unhappy and wants to wait until tomorrow because he feels like he has had enough done to him today, but it really needs to be done to prevent infection. It took a lot of talking to get him to agree; he finally does, but I think he is mad at me. I am only looking out for his best interests, as he seems to get infections easily. I told him that his nurse will give him a nice cocktail (sedative) to make him sleepy and forget, besides, he needs some rest. He has been awake all day and he's tired.

Although the day went well, it was not a happy day for me. Bob was agitated and not happy with what has gone on during the day. He was even upset with me for letting them put in the PICC line. I try to understand that he is on a lot of medication, has been through a lot, and is probably just tired. I still love him a lot, and he knows it.

One of the guys we know from our support group meeting got a heart this morning; we are told he is doing well. We are happy for him.

January 24th, Tuesday. Who knew what today would bring? The day started out with two units of blood because he is very anemic. The doctors did their rounds and said that he is looking a little stronger, probably because he had a good night's sleep. The rectal tube came out last night, so one less attachment. For lunch he was able to have six spoons of tomato soup, two bites of grilled cheese and a quarter cup of milk; doesn't sound like much but he has not eaten for weeks. Progress, is slow and steady.

ECHO was going to be performed this afternoon, because his flows (how the LVAD is pumping blood) are down. Bob may have fluid around his lungs, and has been in a slow decline since 2:00 p.m.; the docs are wondering what is going on. His surgeon is checking on him often and can't figure out why his flows are down, because he has no data to go by – they had removed his Swan and Arterial Line that measure pressures and help them determine what the body is doing.

The Arterial Line and Swan Line are reinserted so they can get more accurate measures as to what his body is doing. He is taken to see if they can drain some fluid from around the lungs; it's 8:00 p.m. and when he is brought back an hour later, they had not done the procedure because there was not enough fluid to drain. I'm staying until they can figure this out.

Doctors are working to get your BP (Blood Pressure) back up and your flows up; something is just not right. I am now scared, but I know they will figure it out. As I wait in the waiting room while they attend to Bob, all I can do is pray, worry and wonder. Please help me, God.

Doctors have been concerned since 3:00 p.m. His breathing is heavy and labored. ECHO is being performed, but this one is where they will go down the throat to see what is happening.

It's about 11:30 p.m. and the surgeon and cardiologist come out to talk to me. They sit down and say, "We have good news and we have bad news. The good news is we found the problem and can fix the problem with Bob's breathing, the bad news is we have to go back into surgery and open him up again to remove a tamponade, which is like a big blood clot pressing against his heart making it hard to breath. If you would sign this consent form we can begin." A nurse came with the form, and I signed. The surgical team has been called in. Another open-heart surgery in the span of three weeks. I was allowed to be with Bob until 1:30 a.m. before he went into the Operating Room.

Not the best day, but not the worst so far. Earlier it was a little bump, now at midnight it is a BIG SCARY BUMP. I feel like I am in an "ER" TV Show - I just can't believe this is happening. I was told it could take a few hours, to go home and I would be called. Home by a little after 2:00 a.m., Jan. 25th, packing and waiting for a call. I was awake until 4:00 and then fell asleep and woke up at 6:45, but no one had called me as I was promised. So I called the nurse and she said the surgery went fine and he was doing well after surgery and got back to the room at 4:00 a.m.

I was very upset, disappointed, and mad that no one called me. Shame on the doctors and Physicians Assistant. I even told them to call my cell number on the board.

January 25th, Wednesday. I arrived back at the hospital at 9:00 a.m. and talked to the PA. He was so sorry - wires got crossed about calling me. I understood, with all the confusion and everyone was tired.

Bob had a massive blood clot pressing on his heart that caused him to decline yesterday afternoon and evening. They think it had been building for some time, because of the size and color. After all that, the surgery went well and now here we go again weaning Bob off drugs and the ventilator once again.

Doctors said that once they opened him up all his numbers went back to normal; it was the pressure causing him problems.

Later today his kidney functions looked better. During

the day he is being weaned off the sedation drugs and hopefully will be awake enough to get off the ventilator.

I ran out to have lunch with Judy and told her the story; she couldn't believe it, what more do we have to endure?

When I returned from lunch Bob was more alert, talking, smiling, wanting water, and he can get off the ventilator at 5:45 p.m.

Bob kept asking me if it was raining, but it wasn't, and then about 6:15 I noticed the floor was wet, really wet. I called the nurse to figure it out and the toilet had overflowed all over the room - boy did they move him rapidly to another room. I guess what had happened was someone on a floor above us had flushed some wipes and they were not to be flushed, oops!! So he heard the running water before we did. Interesting, don't ya think?

Now I know why he was grumpy on Monday and really tired on Tuesday, not wanting to eat or exercise. The pressure on his heart was making him feel that way. We were also told that his breathing was so hard and fast that it was like running a marathon. So lucky he survived, and they found the problem. Sure was another long day; I left early to get some rest after such a long couple of days. Hopefully this is the last of our surprises and surgeries, now onto recovery. Goodnight my love.

January 26th, Thursday. Slept in today because I sure needed it, then went for my morning walk; always clears my head and makes me feel better. When I called, the nurse said that Bob was doing well today. When they moved him last night because of the toilet overflow I forgot to get his glasses, but she told me they found them and Bob has them now.

Arriving at the hospital, Bob said his defibulator

(ICD) shocked him last night; the pacemaker guy came in and made some adjustments. They said that it didn't have to be as sensitive now that he has an LVAD.

The surgeon was in a few times today and said that Bob is doing well, and that he is leaving for a week's vacation. I told him to enjoy it; he really needed it after the last few days. He asked Bob, "How you doing Bob? Your wife really reamed my ass the other night," then added, "That probably was not appropriate." I said, "It's okay, we were all under a lot of stress, and I understand the mix up." I really was more upset with the PA, not Doctor.

My friend Karen and I went to lunch, always a nice break, and then we spent the rest of the day just being quiet and resting.

January 27th. Well, it's finally the end of another long week, and with all that's happened, we are praying for a quiet weekend. Just as I wrote that, the nurse told me that Bob had an incident overnight, which made his central venous pressure (CVP) go up when they were turning him. They put him on a CPAP machine to help his breathing. Bob had the nurse call me at 2:30 a.m. (boy did I jump out of bed, and wide awake as well) to let me know about this. He was very upset, and he thought he was dying and wanted me to come to the hospital. But his nurse said he was fine, and I didn't need to come; he was just scared because he was having a difficult time breathing, and with what he had been through this week, it's understandable, he was frightened. We talked and I told him to remain calm, and that I loved him, and he said, "I love you too."

I finally got back to sleep and woke at 8:00 a.m., called his nurse to see how he was doing; she said they are taking him down for a CT Scan to see if they can drain some fluids. He had a bad night with breathing and they figured there might be fluids around his lungs.

I arrived around 9:30 and we talked about last night. We cried because he was so scared and thought he was going to die. He went down for the CT Scan at 11:00, and I went to lunch with Judy. Bob returned at 1:10 p.m. The procedure went well, and some fluid was drained. Bob was asking for pain medication, as he said the place where they drained fluid was hurting. A quiet day of rest, and he looked a little better in the afternoon. I decided to stay close by tonight so that I didn't have to drive. I am just so tired, and this way I can stay a little later to keep him company. After last night he wanted me to stay longer, so I left at 9:40 p.m. Wow, what a week, probably the most trying week for me so far; a lot of ups and downs.

January 27-28, weekend. I am praying for a nice quiet weekend, and a good night's sleep. I am back at the hospital by 9:30 a.m. Bob is to nap with his CPAP on because he is a little short of breath, and this helps, so they let him use it. During rounds, the doctors talked about the right heart and the meds that are helping support it, and they also said to just get stronger.

Having a quiet day, we went through some of the get well cards he has been receiving. The nurse took the swan line out, also stopped his BP meds and unwrapped his legs. PT and OT were both in, did leg exercises and played with a balloon. Bob seemed to like that activity, and he is quite humorous today; he calls his feeding tube his nose ring, just being funny, must be feeling better. Also worked on deep breathing exercises.

Bob's tummy was upset most of the day, but he did start to use the bathroom, and this made him feel a little better.

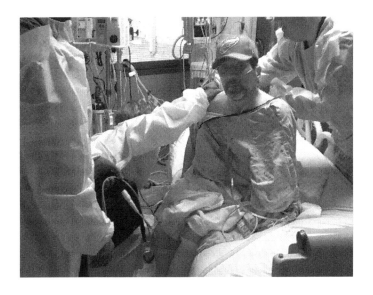

Sitting Up With Help from Physical Therapy

Sunday, PT and OT in for more exercises and therapy, looking bright-eyed and bushy-tailed today. The Sheeans came for a visit, and I went to lunch with them, and when I got back Bob was sleeping. A little better appetite today, so he had beef broth and Italian Ice (liquid diet), we watched golf and relaxed - nice to have a quiet day. A better day today, but still a long road ahead. I left, stopped for gas and a few groceries.

January 30, 2012, Monday. Day 37 in ICU. Most days I try to sleep in, but usually get up by 7:00 a.m., have coffee, go for my walk, get ready, and head for the hospital. Hospital staff keeps reminding me to take care of myself, so I am trying to do that. I know that when Bob comes home I will need to be with him 24/7, so now is my time to get prepared.

When I arrived at the hospital I had to wait in the waiting room, as they were taking out some of Bob's chest tubes, two from surgery. The other two for the lungs have to stay in for a little while longer. When I got to see Bob this morning, I was surprised and happy to see that his feeding tube was gone. Bob said, "I pulled it out last night in my sleep." I was shocked, but the nurse said he took off his Bi-pap mask, pulled the feeding tube out, and put his mask back on. We can't believe you pulled it out; it is about 2 ½ feet long, goes through your nose and into your stomach. Now he has to have another swallow test to make sure no damage was done when he pulled it out.

Well, he passed the test and can have solid food, so he ordered a burger and fries for dinner, but he only ate a few bites; it will take time to get his appetite back. It's funny - he goes from liquid diet to soft food then a burger?? Anyway, he needs to eat and get enough calories and protein, so that he won't have to go back on the feeding tube.

A chest X-ray from where he pulled the tubes was done, and it looked fine.

We trimmed his goatee today, and washed his hair. OT (Occupational Therapy) came for a short time. Bob stood by the bed for a few, maybe 45 seconds (baby steps), then sat down, and then had to get back up to use the commode. I emailed a picture of him sitting on the bed to my sister Sue and his son Derek. My sister emailed back, "Awesome!" So many people are praying and rooting him on to recovery.

January 31, 2012, Tuesday. I got a call from the hospital this morning but no one was there when I answered. This made me a little nervous, and so I called back and the nurse said that Bob wanted to use his Bi-Pap machine and they found it as he was dialing, so he hung up. So many (scary) things were going through my head.

We had a nurse today that we really didn't care for. She may be an excellent nurse, but her bedside manner just doesn't jive with us. I guess this happens when you're here as long as we have been.

Bob had a nosebleed for two hours this morning before it finally stopped. Because of the blood thinners and his LVAD pumping continuously, it takes time to clot; this sure tires Bob out. He asked for something to relax him, because he was all worked up over the nosebleed.

PT and OT came in at 2:00. He sat on the edge of the bed, and stood up and down three times, an improvement from yesterday. PT said he used his own legs to get up with very little help from them. He took a couple of steps to the right, good job, he should be proud of himself. I cried with joy to see him standing; it's been so long.

Lunch was a few bites of stew, ice cream, and sipping on chocolate protein shakes. Not too hungry for dinner, but managed a few bites of lasagna and cake. Bob was worried about the bi-pap machine and wanted to use his own, but they prefer to use the hospital's machine because they can monitor his breathing better, volume, etc. He was okay with that after they explained why. We said our goodnights and I went home.

February 1-3, 2012. Today Bob made a big advancement, and walked out to the sink in the hallway, forty feet. He needed help with a walker, but he was vertical and moving forward, and that's what counts; he hasn't been out of his room in thirty-nine days (on his feet). This was a BIG DEAL!

The next day he walked ninety-eight feet. We were all so happy with his accomplishment, and the third day he walked one lap around the nurses' station, 135 feet. Bob was funny, saying, "I felt like Forest Gump and just wanted to take off." We all laughed, and boy it sure felt good to laugh.

The next few days were working with PT and OT on getting stronger, taking naps, and trying to eat; he still doesn't feel like eating, and just manages small amounts, like a half sandwich, half fruit, half hamburger, half baked potato. It's just going to take time. However he did eat a good dinner of spaghetti one night and said it tasted good; small steps to getting stronger. He likes the protein drink, and that will help.

Had a blood clot in the back of his throat from the nosebleed he had earlier in the week that wouldn't come out. His nurse said it would work its way free - now that's a nice thought.

Judy came for a visit and we went for an appetizer and a glass of wine. A friend of Bob's came for a visit as well. Doctors are happy with his progress, and they said, "YOU have to help us get you stronger," and Bob said, "I'm trying, Doc!"

The last couple of days Bob has had a couple of nurses that he really doesn't care for, so we talked to the floor supervisor and explained our concerns; they will make sure we don't have those nurses in the future. They understand that there are going to be personality conflicts and are willing to work with the patients to make them comfortable. Feeling better tonight on my drive home; small improvements make me feel more at ease.

February 4, Saturday, Day 42 ICU. I'm off for my usual morning walk and routines. When I arrived, Bob had already been to PT and walked 1½ laps this morning, approximately 225 feet. WOW! GREAT JOB!! Bob was very tired and was having a hard time catching his breath. He put his bi-pap machine on and this helps him to catch his breath; probably tired from his walk this morning.

The surgeon was in and he said everything is looking good. Down to one IV, taking out the tube on the right side, and the A-Line (arterial line) is coming out as well. We heard that he may be moved out of ICU and to the cardiac floor, but there are no beds available, and there are twelve patients in line. For now we will stay in ICU and wait.

We then got word at 3:00 p.m. that we are moving, hallelujah! We got moved and settled by 5:30 p.m. Ate a good portion for dinner, and spent the evening watching TV. I left him in good hands, although he was breathing harder when I left. Had to stop for gas and groceries on the way home. I called when I got home and the nurse said he was breathing better. A good day, to get out of ICU after 42 days. It's so much nicer and the rooms are bigger, and I don't have to wait to be announced to get to Bob's room. Yes dear Lord, it has been a good day, thank you!!

February 5, 2012, Super Bowl Sunday! Bob is a much happier guy today - it's Super Bowl Sunday, out of ICU, a bigger room with a window, and of course the nice big screen TV in the room. We spent the day watching golf and then the football game. I went out and picked up a pizza for the game.

We can't forget your PT, when you walked two laps around the nurses' stations (longest walk so far), leg strengthening exercises; he is doing such a good job. A pretty good day all around. Still a long way to go, but an improvement, slow and steady.

February 6-9. The days are now filled with Physical, Occupational, and Recreational Therapy, working on strength. Walked to X-Ray, which is quite a distance, but had to be wheelchaired back, sitting up and out of bed for longer periods of time. Also PT is taking him to the gym to work on machines, like the bike he rode for over seven minutes, leg pumping, walking between rails to help his legs get stronger to get off the walker.

Meds have been lowered and his catheter was taken out. Bob's appetite still isn't great, but at least he gets his protein from protein drinks; food will come with time. Usually an afternoon nap, tired from all the exercising; that's all good.

I met Judy for lunch and I brought back lasagna, although he didn't eat too much; it was probably too heavy anyway. Bob is getting tired of the hospital food, so we try Wendy's chili one night and that tastes good. We will have to figure something out as far as food so he can get good nutrition.

One morning another nosebleed when getting out of bed; ENT (ear, nose and throat doctor) came and inserted a balloon into the nose for pressure to stop the bleeding, and that has to stay in place for a few days.

Another ECHO, which he seems to have often; need to make sure heart is working properly.

We had our first LVAD training class and watched the dressing change. Tomorrow I will do the change with them watching me. I have to be watched and pass the test before I can do it on my own.

Wow, what an experience that is - I did the change today. I was very nervous but did okay. Yucky to see this tube coming out of the body and have to clean around it, it has to be lifted a little, but not too much; it still is not healed and may take some time to heal. I am sure I will learn and be fine with it. One has to do what one's gotta do, right?

Bob had some heavy breathing again, so another chest X-Ray to see if anything is causing this, but it didn't show anything abnormal.

We rest and nap; I get tired too, jumping up and down to help Bob all day long. So when he has a good day, I do too.

February 10-11. We are now in the hospital 49 days. He continues to work out in the gym, walking to the gym or back, but not both. He tries to nap but keeps getting interrupted. One of the doctors said the breathing is the last to come around. He was on and off a ventilator for so long, and the lungs will take time to strengthen and that will get better as he gains strength.

ENT wants to leave the plug in his nose for three more days. We did get his hair washed and a shave, and this made him feel better. He is still so weak that he can't push himself up in bed and he keeps slipping down, so the nurses come in and boost him up, move him, and try to make him more comfortable.

He really isn't feeling well; this is so hard for me to

see him depressed and not up to par. Tomorrow has to be better.

Continuing with OT and PT but tired, so it was cut short. I had LVAD class today, to teach us what to do when we get home. I changed Bob's dressing and went over care for the VAD, and how to change the batteries. I'm tired and need a break, so I go for a walk to get some coffee and fresh air while Bob naps. Still not eating much for dinner; just not hungry. This is so frustrating for me, as he really needs to eat but just doesn't feel like it. We are told it is because of his heart function that he has no appetite.

Walking a little, not long distance, and we take the wheelchair in case he gets tired. Down to the gym, eight minutes on the bike today, increased the resistance on the leg machine, also good improvement with the use of the walker.

ENT came to take the nose plug out, but after looking at it they decided to wait another day; chances of bleeding again still too high; maybe tomorrow.

February 12, 2012, Sunday. Sitting up in a chair when I arrived, he looks better today; that makes me feel better, not so stressed. He ate a good lunch and all of it. Finally his nose plug came out, I'm sure this makes him feel better.

We had a couple of visitors - Sheeans, Terry brought chocolates, and our neighbors, John and Denise. A busy couple of hours and that really tired him out, but happy to see new faces and talk, too. I did the dressing change without a hitch. I think I can do it on my own now. No PT or OT today because of his nosebleed. The docs want to give it time to clot before he starts working out again, so a day off from exercise. Tired after our visitors, we both needed a nap. A quiet rest of the day.

February 13, 2012, Monday. PT had him walk two laps around the nurses' station, plus back to the station and back again to his room. Doctor was in and said, "Keep up the good work, it just takes time."

More friends today, Mike and Paula visited for an hour and half.

Then his blood pressure began to rise, so they had to give meds to help. I notice his blood pressure has been going up since they have been trying to wean him off Dobutamine (medication to help the heart pump). Doctor said it could happen, but it still makes me very nervous; we don't need any setbacks at this point. He had two doses of medication for BP and it is coming down and the flows on the VAD are better at 5:00 p.m. In bed most of the day after PT, now back in his chair for dinner. Overall a pretty good day, he even moved his legs off the bed by himself, usually we have to help swing his legs off the bed. Exercising is paying off.

February 14, Valentine's Day. I had a fun morning dressing in red, and stopping for balloons and a card. When I arrived, people were smiling at me with all the balloons walking through the lobby. Recreational Therapy was in before I arrived, and Bob made me a Valentine Card. It is so cute; I love it and will treasure it forever. Handmade!! WOW.

Just because it is Valentine's Day does not mean he can skip PT, so off to the gym. He rode the bike for ten minutes and was a little tired, so had to be wheelchaired back. Stronger today than yesterday, looking better as well; a little more improvement each day. He is still breathing a little heavy today; doctor ordered a sniff test for tomorrow to see how his diaphragm is working. It's so good to see these baby steps he makes each day; it's a long tunnel and some day we will see the light.

February 15, 2012, Day 53. It's hard to believe that it's been almost two months. Another busy day, PT, and Bob walked to the gym - good job. Sniff test came back normal.

The psychiatrist came to talk, asking lots of questions. The doctors want to see about a sleep medication that is not addictive, and also started him back on Celexa for anxiety. He sat up all day until 3:00 p.m. in a chair. He is acting very anxious and asked for an Adavant for anxiety, but it makes him extremely sleepy and lethargic. For the rest of the afternoon he tried to sleep, but wasn't feeling well; didn't even eat dinner.

It's around 8:00 p.m., and Bob is having a hard time talking and progressively getting worse, the numbers are dropping on his VAD, blood pressure is dropping, and he tells me he is scared, he doesn't know what is happening, and he just doesn't feel right.

I called the nurse, then a nurse from ICU came in; they are trying to figure out what is happening. I am crying and yelling for help, he is just not right, babbling, not making any sense. He last spoke to me at 8:45 p.m. and said, "I Love You, Pammy Poop," (his pet name for me). Then he became unresponsive.

The PA arrived and immediately called for the Blue Bag and began to pump to give him oxygen. I was escorted to the hallway and the code blue team began to show up with the cart, ICU doctors and nurses - it was total chaos.

I was sitting in the hallway, crying and praying to God that he would live. I looked up and the light above his door was blinking BLUE. I asked if that was because he coded and was told yes.

It seemed like hours, but soon our nurse looked around the door of his room and said, "He's okay, we have a pulse." The ICU doctor came to talk to me and asked me if he wanted to go through this again. I said, "What do you mean?" and he said, "Does he want to be brought back again?" Of course he does and I do too!

After that he was taken to ICU, so I cleaned out his room, took things to the car, and went to the ICU waiting room to wait for word of what was happening. His surgeon and his PA came to tell me they are going to do a CT Scan to rule out a stroke, and an ECHO to see what is going on with his heart. It could be a combination of meds, Adavant, thyroid meds, anxiety, his recent labored breathing, etc. They will find out!

When I finally get to see him it is after midnight. He is sedated and on the ventilator again, wrapped in a bubble heater, because his temperature got so low they had to warm him up. His surgeon and cardiologist are in the room, and they asked if I am okay, and will I be able to drive; I said yes. There was nothing else I could do, he was going for testing and he was stable. I told Bob I loved him and would see him tomorrow.

I cried all the way home. I couldn't believe what had happened. Is he going to be okay, live or die, what I am going to do? Made it home, now it was time to try to sleep; I cried myself to sleep once again.

February 16-19. Arriving when the visiting hours start

at 9:00 a.m., the nurse filled me in on the results from last night. The CT Scan was fine, and his numbers are looking good today. It was explained to me that he had too much CO_2 in his blood, which along with the Adavant he took for anxiety and his weakness, all contributed to his becoming unresponsive last night. The Swan line was reinserted, in order to keep a closer eye on his vitals. Bob is sleeping, or should I say sedated again, but he knows I am there. When the sedation drugs wear off they will get him off the ventilator.

By 12:30 he started to wake up, and we had a quiet afternoon. I had lunch with Judy, who told me I looked so tired, and I was.

We did manage to bathe him and change his dressing. Finally at 7:15 p.m. he was awake enough and his vent tube came out. I left at 7:45; he was sleeping and I was so tired, but relieved that he was doing okay.

Next day, the nurse said he has to have another swallow test, but the surgeon said he will be fine; he wasn't on the ventilator that long, and to give him a liquid diet. Bob seems to be breathing better today.

Lynn H. one of Bob's friends came for a short visit.

OT came in the morning, and PT in the afternoon; he managed to walk two laps and sat up in a chair until 3:30 p.m. While he was sitting he had a hot flash, and the flows on his VAD dropped to 2.9. They should optimally run about 4.5. The Perfusionist and doctors came by to see what could have caused this. So, more testing - ECHO, Doppler his legs, all tests came back normal. I decided to stay the night close to the hospital; I was tired and did not feel up to driving.

The next day was not a really good day - tired, upset stomach, just seemed wiped out; did manage a short walk. We tried ginger ale and crackers, a shot of something to help his tummy, but nothing was helping. He did eat a little spaghetti for lunch; that was all. His Dobutamine was increased. He hasn't produced any pee in 4-5 hours, so something is just not right, but what? Trying to figure it out, they are giving extra fluids via IV, still nothing. We'll see what tomorrow will bring. I stayed at a hotel again tonight; just want to be close since Bob has had a tough couple of days.

He is looking better today; the catheter came out last night and he started to pee. Had a better night's sleep, walked two laps even though he still is not feeling well. He was also able to sit up in his chair after his walk. Doctor said the nausea is because his right heart is not functioning like it should; it will take time. We napped most of the afternoon, watched a Red Wings game, then golf. Really bad nausea today.

February 20, 5 days back in ICU. He walked three laps, feeling better than the last couple of days, and also seems to be breathing better. What a relief, not only has it been rough on him these last few days, but I have been stressed, sad, and just wonder when will this turn around, so that we can go home. Overall it was a better day, he ate most of his dinner, exercised, napped, but they can't move him back to the cardiac floor until he is breathing better. So let's pray for better breathing overnight.

February 21, Day 59. Just amazing, so hard to believe we have been here so long. Another nosebleed this morning, packed but not as packed as the last time.

Having a better day today, ate a little stew for lunch; PT waited until the afternoon to walk because of the nosebleed. Did four laps, longest walk so far, great job.

Lunch with Judy again. She is such a great lunch buddy, although she is leaving for Florida for a week tomorrow and I will miss her.

Surgeon was in and said, "Take the Swan Line out, take the A-line out, and let's get him upstairs to the cardiac floor providing there is a room for him." Three hours later we moved out of ICU, yea, happy to be going. Takes time to get him settled and once he is, I decide to go home, praying for a good night.

February 22-29. The next week or so was routine, PT, OT, Recreational Therapy. He is improving and getting stronger, walking longer distances, more reps on the machines in the gym, sitting up more, going to the bathroom on his own but with my help to get there because of the IV Pole and LVAD cords; eating a little better as well. I am changing the dressing every day on my own now, we nap and watch TV.

On Wednesdays we go to the Transplant Support group meetings, where there are people that have had Heart Transplants and others who are waiting, or on LVAD's, and also those that are thinking of a Transplant or going through the evaluation process. It's a great group; we have so much in common to share, and we enjoy getting out of his room.

Since Bob is really getting tired of the food, I decided to start bringing in food from home, and it was approved as long as I stayed low sodium, and a cardiac diet. I can prepare the food at home and then heat it in the microwaves in the cafeteria. Bob is eating better having home cooked meals. Like one day I brought homemade spaghetti, another day baked chicken, sweet potatoes, salad.

Doctors are still adjusting medications, concerned about his fluid retention. It's a balancing act between meds and fluid intake. He has had a few little V-Tachs lately, so he is getting potassium and magnesium, since he has peed a lot and his electrolytes might be off.

Then there are the nosebleeds, nose packed, they wait a few days, he starts bleeding again, and it's packed again, a vicious cycle. It also keeps him from exercising, because that can cause added pressure on the nose, and more bleeds.

Neighbors came for a visit one day. They told Bob he looked good, but later told me that they were surprised by how much weight he has lost and how weak he looked. Weight loss to date is forty pounds, so yes, he has lost a lot, but look what he has been through. I know he will gain weight back. Although it is hard for me to see him this way, we are focused on the end result, a happy healthy heart.

March 1-4, Days 68-71. Started working with Cardiac Therapy, usually they just take him for a walk; it is mainly to see how his breathing is when he is walking. PT takes him to the gym for strength, and OT works with his motor skills.

There are days when we are tired and just nap and then days when we are up and walking more, just taking a day at a time. He had a long walk all the way to X-Ray, which is downstairs, and part of the way back without a walker, but did need a chair to wheel back part of the way.

March 4 blood work shows he is very anemic, so he's getting a unit of blood to help. Also having trouble catching his breath, oxygen levels are good, so it is not that he is not getting enough oxygen. Doctor said to sit up and open your chest to expand your lungs and this will help with your breathing. (Just what I was telling him, but he didn't listen to me.)

A record of his weight, temperature, and other stats are posted on the board in his room, and I just realized that he has lost seventeen pounds in seven days, some of it water but the rest? Eat more and get more protein. Doctor wants him to drink 3-4 protein drinks a day. Bob said, "If I do that, I won't feel like eating." Just do your best, it will come.

Judy is back from vacation; we had a nice lunch while Bob napped. I decided to leave a little early tonight, as I want to make him a special dinner for tomorrow, his birthday.

March 5, Happy Birthday. I bring in balloons, cake, and a nice dinner. During the day the docs do their rounds and say to keep up the good work getting stronger. Works hard in the gym, up to six sets on the Movado machine; it's like doing squats but on a machine where he stands up, three sets at 20% of his weight and three at 25%, then walked back to his room as well.

Birthday lunch is a roast beef sandwich, and the hospital sent up two pieces of chocolate cake with a Happy Birthday sign. We laughed and thought what a nice thing to do.

Good day, he stood at the sink, washed, trimmed his goatee for the first time by himself, another walk with Cardiac Rehab, and then a nice dinner. We had shrimp cocktail, shish kabobs, rice, and cake for dessert. His brother and his son Derek called wishing him a Happy Birthday. A pretty good birthday, feeling better today, and

I am so happy. Who would have thought last Christmas that you would be celebrating your 59th birthday in the hospital, day 72?

March 6-10. The days that follow are busy like most days. ENT doctors had to come again for another nosebleed; this time they used a glue to see if that would help. There was talk of maybe doing a surgery to ablate the veins in the nose. But so far so good, no bleeding, so maybe no surgery. PT in the morning, support group meeting like every Wednesday. He also had his first PFT (Pulmonary Function Test), which checks the lungs to see how well they are progressing in getting stronger. The test showed his lungs are still weak and need improvement. First trip down to the Recreational Therapy room this afternoon to play Hula Hoop on the Wii. I helped Bob get cleaned up, washed hair, bathe with the wipes since he can't get into a shower with the open wound from the cord on the VAD.

Another bump, just a little one, he developed diarrhea. The nurse requested a specimen, it was tested and he has a bacteria called CDIFF. More medication/antibiotics to treat this. This kept PT from working with him today, but Cardiac Rehab did go for a walk with him. Improving daily, more baby steps, slow and steady.

Another visit from Lynn H, since he was in town. Steve and Jan, friends from Tucson, also paid a visit. Finally getting his toenails cut; it's been months. I manage to get them cut without cutting him. If I slipped, he could bleed being on blood thinners, and it would take time to stop. We have success, and it also makes him feel better, and anything to make Bob comfortable.

March 11-16, Days 78-83. Another nosebleed this morning. I & R is high at 4.1 (measures how well your blood clots - the higher the number the longer it takes to clot), it should be in a range of 2.5-3.0. They are going to give him some plasma to help with his INR; it also could be caused from the antibiotic he is getting. His vitals are being checked more often today because of the plasma.

We managed a walk; he has progressed to walking the "long loop." We call it that because it goes out into the lobby by the elevators to the other wing of the hospital and back again, three long laps complete.

More visitors, the Wyman's, come by. We had a nice visit; they told us how concerned people are at the mine, how everyone asks about him. It's nice to know that many people are concerned.

The rest of the week was routine, PT, OT, Cardiac Rehab, increasing the reps and weights, all good signs of getting stronger, working on getting home. Still a ways to go, but it relieves me to see improvement, and also to see him doing a few things for himself.

Bob's hemoglobin is low which makes him tired, so we nap. Getting his hemoglobin higher will take time as his nutrition gets better and he gets stronger.

A few more visitors this week, as well. Jim was in town from Colorado, John and Denise stopped by for a nice visit. John thought Bob was looking so much better than the last time he saw him, and was relieved to see improvement.

Another nosebleed this week. Of course it was packed again; this will stay in for about five days.

Attended the Support Group meeting on Wednesday.

Always a good meeting to see how others are progressing, and giving support for those waiting for a heart and also those deciding if they want to get an LVAD, and of course good to see those that have had a Transplant and are getting along so well.

His surgeon was in and wanted to see his site where the cord comes out, so when I did the dressing change, he peeked in and said it was slow in healing, but looks good. The LVAD nurse came by as well. Talked about attaching a sponge vac to the site to help it heal quicker, but I think they are going to wait awhile for that. It would just be another machine to carry around and we really don't need that. Healing is slow because of nutrition - so much depends on good nutrition, that's why it's so important to eat well and get enough protein to promote healing. But there are times when Bob just doesn't feel like eating, so he continues with his protein drink. I still bring food from home and heat it up in the cafeteria, in hopes that Bob will want to eat.

March 16 was our first training session to learn how to change over from one controller on the LVAD to another in case one stops working. Really scary because you only have a short amount of time to switch over, and during the time you are switching over, the pump stops working and blood flow stops. Hopefully we never have to switch over.

March 17-20, Days 84-87. St. Patrick's Day. Wow, almost three months. Dressing changes are going to be twice a day for a while to promote healing and ward off infection. More therapy sessions today. Kind of a quiet day and that's okay, usually we are so busy.

I spoke to the mother of a girl waiting for a heart

who said today may be her day. It's 3:00 p.m. and she said surgery was scheduled for 5:00 p.m.

She did get a heart last night and is doing well. We are happy for her; she has waited a long time. We have met a few patients waiting for a heart or recuperating from other surgeries; they too need to get stronger so they can get on the Transplant List. I have become friends with their spouses or family members that are at the hospital as much as I am. We visit each other, we cry together when we have setbacks, supporting each other. It sure helps when you know you're not alone. Some have it better than we do and others have it a lot worse.

Bob is a little short-winded today; it may be because of lowering Dobutamine, which helps his heart pump better. It's a rainy and cold day. Getting up from the sitting position is improving, he's not as shaky in the hands, and he even cut his own steak tonight at dinner. So, little improvements, still baby steps, but they are steps and we can't ask for anything more.

Doctors are talking about moving Bob to another floor where they concentrate on Rehab. The doctor came from the Rehab to evaluate Bob but said he is doing well enough and didn't need to go there.

Had a good workout with PT, then OT had him lifting and getting things from the closets, up and off the toilet, just daily activities that he would be doing at home. He walked for Cardiac Rehab. With the therapy sessions it was another busy day.

March 21. Bob called me on my way in to the hospital and asked me to buy some peppermint candies; he has an upset stomach, and the nurse gave him something for it, but he thought the mints might help too. Had a short PT session and cancelled OT since he was not feeling well. He was sleeping when I arrived and slept until 12:45 p.m.

We went to the Support Group meeting and when we came back, the doctors put him back on Dobutamine again. They are concerned that his upset stomach is because of heart function, and his breathing is also a little labored as well. Did manage to walk to X-Ray and back, so that was good, sat up for about an hour and then back to bed for an afternoon nap. Sat up to eat dinner, and then back to bed. Having a little anxiety when I left, just a tired day and not feeling well. Let's pray tomorrow will be better. I go home and worry, but just another rough day. Called the nurse before I went to bed and she said he was doing a little better and sleeping.

March 22-26, Days 89-93. When I arrived, Bob was outside walking with PT, getting a bit of fresh air and sunshine. Feeling better today, maybe it's the Dobutamine. If he does not start to feel better soon, more tests, like an ECHO, right heart cath etc., to see what is going on with his heart since he had a couple of bad days.

I left early to meet Judy and Carol for dinner and a girls' night out. Sure do need this after the last three months. Had a fun time at the casino with the girls. Didn't win, but it was nice to get out and get my mind cleared out while he is being cared for. I won't be able to leave him alone when we get home, so this was a nice break for me.

The next few days were busy with routine therapy sessions. On Sunday the doctors were thinking of doing an ECHO while he is on Dobutamine and then again when he is off to see the difference in the heart function. Another PFT test this coming week and possible talk and evaluation about getting him back on the Transplant List - just a "maybe" at this point.

They decided later that Bob needs to get home, go to outpatient Cardiac Rehab for twelve weeks, then another evaluation to get back on the list. It was a happy thought for a short time thinking he may get back on the list, but we understand that Bob has to be stronger first, in order to go through another surgery.

Attended an LVAD Support Group meeting; about fifteen people attended. These are the people that are living with the VAD that Bob has, what they call a bridge to Transplant VAD, where he just has the VAD to support his heart while waiting for a donor heart. Learned different ways to wear the VAD equipment. Was a good meeting for us to learn how to live with it for the next few months and to visit with others that will live with it for the rest of their lives.

Another chest X-Ray today, walked to and back. He seems to have more good days than bad lately; it's great to see. He said he can taste more and feels like he's getting some of his appetite back, also good news.

March 27-29, Days 94-96. Another ECHO today since Bob has been off Dobutamine, and a PFT this afternoon. Results on the PFT were about the same as last time, which is not what the doctors are looking for - they want to see improvement. He needs to work with his breathing tool more often to strengthen the lungs. Frustrating for me not seeing improvement, as improvements need to be made so we can go home.

Usual routine with therapy, weights, and walking continues. Neighbors John and Denise came for a visit, and

Candy, my friend from Santiago, Chile, arrived around 3:00 p.m. She is here to help her daughter plan for her wedding in December. Great to see her; she will be staying with me for a few days, and happy to have her company.

March 29. Bob had a right heart cath; results came back normal. Doctor said looking good, now it's time to plan an outing. Wow, what a nice surprise, it means we may be going home; we are both so happy that the time has come after 96 days.

We talked about going to clean out his work office while he is still in the hospital, since he would not be able to travel when he gets out. We agreed that I would make the trip tomorrow and pack his office; I called some friends to help me with that.

Went for lunch with Candy, stopped by a few golf shops, arrived at the hospital about 2:00 p.m.; needed to spend time with her since she is only here for a short time.

Bob not feeling well, upset stomach, doesn't feel like eating, tired. I went home worried that he is coming home in this condition, and how am I going to handle him by myself? Candy and I had a glass of wine and talked way into the night; I cried because I am so scared for Bob to come home after all this time. I will be totally responsible for him, his machine, what happens if the alarms go off or it stops working - all these things are going through my head. I really am nervous. Felt good to share my fears with someone close.

March 30. Left home at 8:00 a.m., traveled north for an hour and a half to pack up Bob's office; Kirsten and Debra helped pack and load the boxes into my car. Finished about 12:30, ate a little lunch, back home by 2:30, at the hospital by 3:45. Bob was napping and still feeling lousy, doesn't know what to do, can't eat, just having a bad day.

When I got home, I couldn't find a file Bob asked me to look for and I am upset about that. It's midnight and I can't sleep, don't know what to do. Tired and frustrated about the situation and life. I want our life back, and with Bob feeling sick it makes me upset that I can't help. Praying tomorrow will be better.

The next day, March 31st, Debra and Richard came to help me load Bob's office boxes into our storage unit, and then I went to the hospital. When I arrived, Bob was in bed; heart rate up and flows on his LVAD are down. They are giving him fluids, thinking he may be a little dehydrated.

It's noon and his heart rate is still high, this really is making me nervous. The EP doctor came to see what might be going on, talked about an oblation to the AV node. Will eliminate the electrical communications between the atrium and ventricle, then the pacemaker will be pacing the heartbeat solely, which would steady the heart rate. The doctors will decide what to do and when.

Had a nice visit from Candy, her three children, Gretchen, David, Harry, and another girlfriend, Thonda, from Mexico. They had been to a baseball spring training game, but took the time to come and visit; so great to see them. They brought Bob a putting green he can use in the hospital and at home to help with his recovery, and a faith-based golf book.

Still having strange heartbeats all day, but feeling better tummy wise. Ate dinner I brought from home - baked chicken and sweet potato.

April 1-3, 2012. Sunday, Day 99. Can you even imagine

ninety-nine days in the hospital? I drive back and forth every day, forty-five minutes each way.

I helped Bob get cleaned up and in his own T-shirt for the first time. PT this morning, lunch, and then we took a walk. Charlie and Debbie paid a visit, then another walk outside for fresh air and sunshine for about half an hour.

Later in the day the cardiologist informed us not to worry about the arterial fibrillation (easy for him to say); it is not hurting him and they really don't want to do anything invasive like an oblation. Sounds like they want to get him home, to get stronger and healthy.

Bob started looking for his cell phone, and we can't find it; we look everywhere, and it's just not around. Then Bob said, "The other night, I heard something drop when I hit the tray table in my sleep and maybe it fell into the garbage can that was below the tray." OOPS!! One lost cell phone. I was sick - can you imagine all those contacts, pictures, emails, gone? We hadn't done a backup in months. Well, we will try to recoup the information at a later time. It's in the landfill by now, I am sure of it. So I guess we will get a new one when he gets home.

Went for take-out for dinner. I just hate to take the time to cook at home if he is not going to eat, plus sometimes I just need a break from cooking every night.

The next couple of days more PT, also walked to the Recreation room with Cardiac Rehab nurse, played baseball on the Wii; something new to do and Bob has enjoyed playing. This activity helps improve balance and strengthen the core. More leg exercises, and changes in some meds for high blood pressure.

Magnesium is borderline at 1.8, so he's getting IV

magnesium, but this in turn causes flows to come down, and the surgeon doesn't like that. I'm sure they will get it figured out. Flows start to improve, also changed a med to Coreg 3.25 mg.

Time to have our outing with the LVAD Coordinator tomorrow. We are so happy but also very nervous. I go home and get the house ready for our inspection tomorrow.

April 4, 2012, Wednesday, Day 102. The big day has arrived! The LVAD coordinator takes us on an outing to see our home. She wants to check our layout, safety, location of where we would put the monitor for the VAD, outlets, electrical box, etc. She explained to us that if there were to be an electrical outage, our home is on a special list to make sure they get the power back on ASAP. Although there are batteries to keep the pump working, it's a precaution. Our outing started out at 11:00 a.m., then we all three went for lunch, and returned to the hospital around 3:00 p.m. That was a long day. They like to see how we will manage being out of the hospital with the new device. So tired that we both took a nap, had a little dinner, and then I left, since we needed groceries for the homecoming tomorrow.

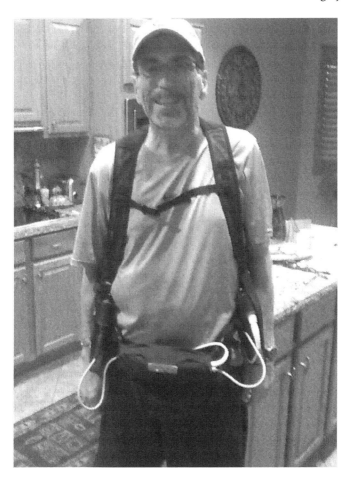

Bob Home With LVAD

April 5, 2012. Thursday, Day 103. Joyous Day, thank you Lord! After one hundred three days in the hospital Bob is finally coming home. We had our last outing by ourselves. We were a little nervous being on our own, even though they told us to take our time and see how it feels. We only went for lunch as we had a busy day ahead

55

with doctors, nurses, social worker and people coming by to wish us well. (We got to know a lot of people when we were there for so long.)

Bob was discharged at 4:15 p.m., we were home by 5:00, I unloaded the car and we relaxed with a simple dinner - burger patty and salad. We are both so tired and happy to be home. Bob just looks around and walks around the house taking it all in. He is happy to see our kitties and they him. I get the equipment set up fine, also the handicap rail for the toilet seat. Finally home sweet home, good night.

April 6, 2012. GOOD FRIDAY, Day 1 at home. We have to go back for an appointment already. The policy is to see the patient three days after discharge but since three days would be a Sunday, we have to go back today at 10:00 a.m. Blood work, LVAD coordinators check the dressing change, they check on us, we have only been home less than twenty-four hours, but it is policy.

Blood work looked good, surgery site is almost healed, and soon Bob can take a shower; that's another chore that I can get into later. We make another appointment for Monday. Back home we have lunch, then relax with a nice nap, watched golf and then hockey. My friend Karen brought by an Easter lily. That was so nice and I love fresh flowers. So great to be home.

April 7-10, 2012. Day 2 at home. The day started out pretty good, had breakfast, and rested most of the day. I cleaned and did laundry, just the usual home chores. About 4:30 p.m. Bob's ICD fired; he was just sitting on the couch and we were resting and waiting for dinner to finish in the oven. We called the VAD Hotline, as instructed if anything out of the ordinary happened, and this was definitely out of the ordinary. After talking to the coordinators and doctor, we were told to come into the Emergency room. Damn, here we go again.

The usual blood work, checked LVAD and ICD. Blood work looked good, but he was admitted back into the hospital. Everyone was so surprised and saddened when we arrived back in the Cardiac Unit; we just left two days ago.

The next day the doctor was in and said Bob had arterial flutters all day yesterday before the ICD fired; again more talk about doing oblations, also another ECHO. He was feeling pretty good today other than very tired, as am I. EP doctor came in; he is going to increase his Amiodrone to 400 mg per day for a month and make some changes to his ICD. An oblation would be the last resort.

We had a good cry, upset that we are back in the hospital. I am trying to be encouraging. Tried to keep busy, shaved, washed hair, and went for a walk. Since we didn't have dinner at home the other night, I brought it in and we enjoyed ribs and potato salad.

Another day went by and we still haven't heard if and when we are going home. Doctor said it is up to the EP doctor; we are wondering what the plan is but no one seems to know. Maybe they are trying to figure it out as well. Went to the cafeteria for dinner. Judy stopped by and brought a glass of wine for her and me. I guess we will wait another day.

April 10. It is decided that we can go home, but before we do, Bob gets a unit of blood to help his hemoglobin. Then we can go home, so we are happy once again. What a roller coaster this week has been. Got his blood unit started at 1:45 p.m., and finished at 4:30. Now that we are going home, the PA is working on our discharge papers, and then we will be out of here!! Yea.

Started to pack up our things and get ready to leave, when Bob had an episode of V-Tach that was detected on the heart monitor in the nurse's station. The PA said that we have to stay. You have got to be kidding. But of course it is not safe for Bob to go home if he is having irregular heartbeats, only to have to turn around and come back. We are extremely disappointed. The PA tells us it's another bump in the road. If I hear "another bump in the road" one more time I am going to scream!!! We are both unhappy, we cry, we just want to be home and start rehab, get stronger and get a heart. Very disappointing day.

April 11-14. Days 108-111 total in the hospital. V-Tach and a fast heart rate kept him from going to Cardiac Rehab in the morning. The cardiac team decided to do the oblation for the AV node to stop the fluttering, which should help with the ICD detecting it as V-Tach, and hopefully he won't get shocked. They wanted to do the procedure this afternoon, but no one told us not to eat, so now it has to wait until tomorrow. Our nurse should have informed us; Bob is not happy that he has to wait because he ate.

We asked to speak to the heart coordinator about a few things, one being the incident about eating, another the nurse forgot to up the blood drip yesterday, so it took longer than it should have, and blood draws were done when they should have waited until after the blood was finished dripping. This has happened before and shouldn't. Also his bed linens had not been changed for a couple of days. I know these seem like little things and not life threatening, but when you are in the hospital as long as we have been, we notice these things. She listened to our concerns and said they would be addressed, and thanked us for letting her know.

April 12. I arrived at the hospital at 9:30 in case they took Bob for his oblation procedure early. It is scheduled for noon, although they could come anytime to get him prepped. One of his surgeons came in and said, "This is a good procedure for you. It will help with your V-Tach. You will be totally dependent on your pacemaker, but then again, you are now." This made us feel good about the procedure, it is the best thing to do, and when we get home we will have one less worry about the ICD firing.

They came for his AB Node oblation at 1:30, to the Cath lab first, then for the procedure at 2:40 p.m. At 3:10 the doctor said all went well, no problems, got in and done the first time. I was able to see him at 4:30 in recovery, and back to his room by 5:15. After this type of procedure where they go through your groin you must lay flat and still for six hours, so no moving until 9:15 p.m.

April 13. A quiet day, an ECHO, walked, not much going on. They increased the heart rate on his pacemaker from 80 to 100 beats per minute to help his flows on his VAD, since they are lower than the VAD doctors would like to see.

April 14. Doctor said one more day to make sure his latest CDIFF is gone and to just watch him. His CDIFF is gone, but his flows are up and down. We walked, napped, and had a nice dinner from PF Chang's, overall a quiet day. Hopefully we can go home tomorrow.

April 15-19, 2012. Sunday, 112 days in hospital total.

We headed home, stopped for lunch and got home by 2:45. So happy to be home once again, let's pray we stay here for a while. The next few days we relaxed; I had my annual mammogram and blood work, Bob got a haircut, and we got caught up on sleep and house chores. We are happy and content being home.

April 17. We go for Bob's check up appointment; all looks good. LVAD coordinators changed his antiseptic; the one we use now is causing a rash. When we got back into our car I said, "They let us out?" We laughed, seems like when we go for an appointment, we end up staying.

The next couple of days were good. Outpatient rehab facility called, and we made an appointment to start cardiac rehab next Tuesday & Friday at 10:30 a.m. Cleaned house, went for small walks around the neighborhood, changed out the screens to sun shades for summer, cleaned the patio, all the things I haven't been able to do for months. Gave Bob a pedicure, Bob used his weights, watched TV hockey, had a nice dinner; living life and enjoying being at home, working our way forward.

April 20, 2012, Friday. Went for a follow-up appointment at noon; doctors didn't like that Bob is retaining more fluids. An ECHO was ordered to check his right heart function. While waiting for the results, one of the LVAD coordinators came out and told us his right heart function is low, and probably this is causing him to retain fluids. The doctors want to admit him. They will put him on an IV medication (Milrinone) to help his right heart function.

We are sad and I began to cry, when will this end? He

may have to go home with this new medication, so that he can have more energy to go through rehab. If it helps him to get stronger and have more energy it will be okay.

Once settled into his room, I drove home to get his Bi-Pap machine and a few other things like clothes and bathroom items to get him through a few days. I called the rehab facility where he has appointments this week and cancelled. The rest of the day was quiet.

April 21-25, 2012. Days 115-118 in the hospital. Bob seems to be feeling better today, more energy, walking without stopping and in good spirits. How he does this I don't know, in and out of the hospital, IV's, PICC lines, everyone poking at him, waking him in the night etc. You know what hospitals are like; you just can't get the rest needed. But he manages with good spirits; he just says whatever it takes to get him well, because he still has a lot of living to do.

When the doctors did their rounds, they indicated that Bob would have to go home on this IV Medication, or rehab here in the hospital on the rehab floor; the team will discuss a plan this week. Well, they don't meet until Wednesday and this is only Saturday, so I guess we will be here for more than a few days.

Continued with PT, OT, Recreational Therapy and cardiac rehab, walking as much as possible, napping, just biding time until they decide what the plan of action is. Another PFT Test, and chest X-Ray. We asked about going home, but no one knows.

Wednesday came, and the surgeon indicated that they would discuss Bob in their Transplant meeting. He said, "I'm pulling for you to get back on the list," but then another doctor said no, he has to go to rehab and get stronger before we put him on the list; also they need to get him out of here to do that. Went to the support group meeting, walked, and washed his hair. Home health care came by kind of late in the afternoon, so probably not going home today, although we were so hoping it would be today.

April 26, 2012. Bob has been in the hospital one hundred nineteen days this year. Let's pray no more until his Transplant. Bob is looking stronger, had a good workout in the gym with PT.

The surgeon came in and said that he must get stronger to handle the Transplant. If his lungs are not strong enough after surgery, they can't take him off the ventilator and he could get an infection, because of the anti-rejection meds he would be on. So, work hard to get stronger. He could tell we were disappointed, and then he sang the tune from <u>Annie</u>, "It's a hard knock life, no it's a Washnock life." We laughed, he is so nice, we like him a lot. He added, "Go home; rehab, get stronger, and I don't want to see you until transplant." We said, "Okay doc!"

Yea, we are going home, but have to wait for home health care to deliver the meds we need to take with us. It took them until 6:30 p.m., who knows what took so long. They knew yesterday we might go home today; it's all so frustrating. Anyway, we got to go home, finally arrived home at 8:00 p.m., exhausted and with a headache.

April 27-29, 2012. It's great waking up at home with Bob beside me, although I don't sleep very well, checking on him to make sure he is breathing. If he wakes up I do too, to make sure he gets to the bathroom, although he uses a urinal at night beside the bed as a safety precaution. This way we don't have to worry about all the cords and the machine in the middle of the night.

I had a doctor's appointment and then we went grocery shopping. The nurse from Home Care came by to check Bob's vitals, and to make sure we knew how to change the IV medication bag. She is really nice and helpful. Now time to relax.

The next day I kept myself busy, washed two cars, cleaned the house, the usual chores. Bob is very tired; he napped on and off all day. We both took the day off from exercising, no pushing him if he is tired.

Talked to our neighbors Charlie and Debbie about going out for brunch with them tomorrow, since they will be leaving for Canada for the summer.

We went for brunch at a little place close to home, had great omelets and a Bloody Mary (well, not Bob.) He is feeling better each day, finally getting caught up on sleep. Our usual afternoon, changed his site dressing, changed his IV Bag, watched TV, took a little walk down the block.

April 30, 2012. Wow, what a day. It started out fine - up early, I went for my walk before Bob got out of bed. I walk just around the neighborhood, not too far away, in case he calls and needs me. Bob got up at 7:30, had breakfast, got washed up (he can do this by himself now.) I decided to do a Real Estate class online for my continuing education classes, since this year is flying by and I need to get a certain number of hours before the end of the year.

Bob was sitting at the dining room table making phone calls to friends and people at work, letting them know how he is doing. I could see him from the office where I was and he's getting up, turns and loses his balance and falls, hitting one of the bar stools at the counter; scared me probably more than him.

I rushed over and checked his controller; it's working. I get him up and we go and connect to the main controller in the bedroom to make sure his numbers are where they should be. I call the VAD Hotline to speak with the coordinator, and told her what happened. She asked if he hit his head, and I said no. I think we are all right now, just shook us up. The rest of the day was quiet, home care nurse came and did her usual vitals, checking his PICC Line. I did a little ironing while Bob napped. Dinner, watched hockey and TV; nice quiet evening at home.

May was a busy month, with going to Rehab three days a week, back and forth with follow-up appointments at the clinic for blood work, checking the LVAD device. They also just like to see how Bob is progressing. We like to eat out for lunch when we have these appointments, although it's hard to find low sodium food when eating out. We manage to have really low sodium on the days we eat at home.

There was one morning when Bob wanted to go out and get the paper from the driveway by himself, so of course I let him go, and wouldn't you know, he lost his balance and fell backwards. I went running out, "Are you okay, are you okay?" He said, "Yes, I'm okay." John, our next-door neighbor, happened to be outside and helped me get him up, since his legs are still very weak.

Once we settled down from the excitement and Bob felt fine, we went to the Social Security office to apply for disability. Bob won't be going back to work for a long time;

he has to get back on the Transplant list, and once he does get the transplant, then there is the recuperation time. We are probably looking at least another year, if not more.

Finally got through all the paper work, and Bob had to use the restroom. At home we have a handicap toilet, which is higher and he can get off that, but if a handicap stall is not available in public he can't get off the toilet because they are too low. He was in there for a long time, so finally I found a man to help me check on him, and he was just sitting there waiting for someone to come in and help him up. If you recall, he lost his phone in the hospital months ago, and has not replaced it. We need to get him a phone, so that if he has a problem he can call me and I can either go in and help or send help. A lesson learned.

We have heard stories from others in the hospital when they applied for disability that it took months to get a response. I guess we were one of the lucky ones, because within a couple of weeks we were approved. Between Social Security, Disability, and his long-term disability insurance through work, we will be okay financially. Others we know didn't have it so good, so we consider ourselves very fortunate.

The Home Care nurse came Monday, Wednesday and Friday, with Rehab on those days as well. Bob got additional exercise walking around the grocery stores, and we took a walk around the block on the days that he didn't have rehab. If it is too hot, we would go to our gym. He is working really hard to get stronger; this is what it is going to take.

My girlfriend Candy returned to help her daughter with wedding plans again, so we had them over for dinner one night, such a nice evening. We have known Gretchen since she was a "pea in the pod," so it was great to meet her betrothed.

Bob woke one morning and his IV meds had leaked all over the bed, so we had to figure out what to do. His line was leaking, so I changed it for a new one, and put a new bag of meds on and it worked out fine. He may have lost a little infusion over the night, but otherwise he was fine.

May 16, 2012. Our usual follow-up appointment. His site was healed well enough, so Bob will be able to shower, great news.

He had developed an itchy rash around his dressing area, so we showed it to doctors and they said to take Benadryl, as he may be allergic to something. Well, Benadryl will make most people sleepy, but not Bob - he was awake, very agitated and thrashing around in bed all night. Neither of us slept well. Little did we know this would happen.

When I woke him, there was blood on the sheets from where his PICC Line is; not a lot, but still a little bit unnerving. It was probably due to his restlessness all night. Cleaned up the blood, checked his PICC line and everything looked fine. We were tired from last night and decided not to do much today, other than go to Rehab.

May 17 was a momentous day. Bob took his first real shower in about one hundred forty days. We were given a specially made bag to hold his LVAD controller, and we wrapped his arm where his PICC Line is with special waterproof tape and a plastic sleeve. I got into the shower with him so that he doesn't slip and I can help him wash. Tight quarters, but we manage. Bob said, "Oh that felt soooo good." Our next goal is for him to shower by himself, although there is no hurry, all in good time.

The rest of the month we went out for brunch with friends Karen and Terry, and Bob's son Derek and his wife, Alicia drove from Salt Lake City to visit for a few days; we truly enjoyed their visit. Although we didn't (couldn't) do too much, it was nice to have them visit.

Tuesday after Memorial Day, another follow-up appointment, and a nurse changed Bob's dressing. Still itchy, so a decision was made to change to a type of dressing that will let a little more air to the area. Also the LVAD Coordinator is helping with finding a place to buy the dressing changes, in order for the insurance to cover the cost. Otherwise it is $200.00 a month just for those supplies. She is looking into insurance coverage of a holster vest for Bob's equipment as well. They scheduled another PFT (Pulmonary Function Test) for June 26, to see the progression of the lungs.

June 2012 was a good month. We both had our eyes checked and got new glasses, Bob continued with Rehab and is almost complete - he will be graduating from Cardiac Rehab soon. I can see little improvements in his strength, his voice is sounding more like him, and the rash is clearing up, so lots of positive things happening.

The insurance approved the dressing change supplies, also a new vest to hold Bob's equipment, the batteries and controller. We are happy because the new vest will make it easier for Bob is get around and also help with his balance.

Bob had a kidney test, and his PFT came back base line, great news, this means his lungs are getting stronger. Bob was so happy about the PFT; he is different, happy and really looking forward to getting a new heart. Our lives are changing. We really don't remember what it is like to be normal (like we were before his heart problems), 14 years, now we will be able to start anew. Waiting on the results of the kidney test. If all is good, he may get back on the Transplant List.

While we were at the hospital one day for an appointment, we paid a visit to a patient we knew when Bob was there. He is still working on a number of medical issues that are keeping him from getting on the list, but he is trying so hard. We also paid a visit to ICU to see Bob's favorite nurse; so many of the staff were happy to see Bob and how well he is doing.

July turned out to be another busy month. Bob had a new Medic-alert bracelet made, with a Southwest style. He has finished with outpatient Rehab, so now we go to the gym to continue his exercising. We had lunch with friends and went to the movies - a "normal" life while carrying around this machine in a pouch on his side.

At our last appointment there was still some concern about Bob's kidney function, so we are going to see the kidney doctor, and go through testing for his kidneys. This is to make sure that his kidney function is what it needs to be before he goes on the list, in case he needs a kidney as well as a heart. The medications taken after transplant can lessen kidney function, so they want to make sure his can handle the medications. His kidney function should get better with a new heart, however.

The kidney function test is scheduled for the 10th, at 1:00 p.m., no eating four hours prior to the test and the test could take three hours. I feel sorry that he can't eat for so long, but at least we are getting these tests done and Bob can get back on the transplant list sooner. Just have to wait for the results, and once the Transplant team gets the results and talks to the kidney doctors, they can decide.

Bob is doing really well, stronger each day and working hard at his in-home rehab, and progressing. However, his ICD went off at 7:45 p.m. on the 15th, which always scares us because you never know if it will go off again. We called the VAD hotline, and were told as long as there are no symptoms and flows are good, to stay home and come in the morning for a checkup.

More appointments, blood draws and ECHOs as well, also they want to do another right heart cath, to check the function of the right heart; it is scheduled for 2:30 p.m. The procedure went well; numbers were good, although his Amiodorone is being increased to 800 mg for a week, then back to 400 mg per day. No exercising for the rest of the week. We thought because of his ICD firing we may end up in the hospital again, but they let us go home.

Arriving home, Bob couldn't find his wedding ring, he may have lost it in the men's room; we called lost and found to report it in case someone finds it. We are both sick that he may have lost his ring.

During the night his right heart cath site began to bleed, not badly, but there was blood present; we were awake a few times in the night changing the bandage, and we managed to stop the bleeding.

Dermatology appointment for 8:00 a.m. on the 18th, to check out the rash on his legs. We decided to go over the night before as to not have to deal with traffic. It was interesting, packing all the batteries for the LVAD,

Melrinone supplies for his IV, etc. We managed just fine although I was nervous, since it is the first overnight away from home.

While getting ready, Bob wore the shorts he was wearing on the day he lost his ring and voila, there was his ring deep in the pocket. We are so happy, and he said, "I always put my ring in my pocket when I wash my hands. I didn't think I would have left it in the bathroom." His hands are so small now that I thought maybe it had fallen off. Anyway, we are glad he found it. Got to the hotel at 7:45, settled in and watched TV.

It is also Wednesday, when the Transplant Team meets to decide if Bob will make the list. No news today, so I guess we have to wait another week. Appointment at the dermatologist went fine, they took a biopsy of the rash and it will be tested, and they suggested a cream to use.

The next week of waiting consisted of more exercises, buying groceries, the usual, but then on Wednesday night we found a bump on his neck where the right heart cath was done ten days ago. It looked like blood, so we will see what it looks like in the morning.

The bump looked the same, and our Home Care nurse wasn't sure either. We decided to call the VAD hotline and the coordinator asked us to come in. We were going in on Friday anyway to get the stitches out from the biopsy of the rash, so we went in for them to check it out.

While we were at the appointment Bob had some odd heartbeats, couldn't figure it out. His flows came down on the VAD machine, so he drank some water - maybe he is dehydrated. When the pacemaker nurse came in, his heart rate was back to normal, but I was nervous at this point, wondering what is going on. After drinking water, the flows came back up, but they still want to do an ECHO this afternoon.

We decided to go out for lunch while we waited for the ECHO appointment. While having his ECHO the VAD Nurses, Perfusion came, all checking Bob out. Everything seemed to be okay, just told us to make sure Bob drinks enough water. He was taken off Lasix, which is a medication for fluid retention, and told to take it only as needed.

July 26, 2012, it's 6:00 p.m. and we get a phone call from the Transplant Coordinator informing us that Bob is back on the Transplant list, a 2-B status. Wow, what a day - we went in for stitches to be removed, and to check the bump on his neck, and then this happened. We are elated, and now we wait for the phone to ring. It truly is a GREAT DAY. I am a little scared - another surgery, although I know it is what needs to happen, it is scary. After meeting other Heart Transplant recipients we know it will be okay, back to living life, golf, travel etc. We have two hours to get to the hospital after we receive the call that a heart is available, so we wait with bags packed.

August, we continue with doctor appointments for check-ups. One day while we were at an appointment we ran into one of the Transplant surgeons, who told us that Bob is moving up on the list, and to keep our phone close and that Bob was looking good. We go on with life, changing IV bags, dressing changes, exercising, groceries, and all the usual things.

At one appointment it was decided to lower Bob's Melrinone, and switch him to an oral medication. They would like to wean him off the Melrinone, which would take a couple of weeks, so he could then be taken off the IV pump, since the IV area is just another area that could develop infection. He will be monitored closely for signs of water retention, shortness of breath, etc. Otherwise he is doing well.

Also we are educated on the medications he would be on after Transplant and we need to learn both the name and also the generic names. The sooner the better, we are told. So we begin to learn them and what they are for, also what they look like; we will be quizzed at our next appointment.

A couple of days later we received a call from our VAD coordinator informing us they are taking Bob off the Melrinone and will be given a new drug call Revatio, to help his heart and lungs. Not too happy about this, since we don't know that much about this drug, but after talking to a nurse from the doctor's office, we feel better about taking the drug.

A few days later Bob started Revatio, keeping him on his IV Med as well. Went to a matinee movie with Terry and Karen, and then had them over for dinner since it was Terry's birthday. A good day, good movie, good dinner and friends. Such a busy Saturday, so Sunday was a day to relax and watch the Olympics.

August 13-19. Home Care nurse came over to check on Bob, we went to the gym, did things around the house, ironing etc. a pretty quiet day. I did get a little upset when Bob wanted to take a nap before we went to the gym. I guess what set me off was on his way to take a nap he said he needed a glass of water, and he couldn't get it because he needed to go to the bathroom. Well, go to the bathroom and then get your own water is what I thought; he can do things for himself, but still relies on me for everything. I have no time for myself. I haven't been away from Bob for months. It's all about him and I know that it is, but I feel l need some time for myself. Just feeling a little trapped right now, I know I will get over it. I am just venting.

Tuesday, another good appointment. One doctor wants to change his Melrinone, another said why rock the boat, he is doing well, just keep it as it is, and they will discuss what treatment will be the best for him Wednesday.

We never heard of any changes so we continue as we have with the meds. Bob had a few restless nights with itching, peeing etc.

It's now the end of August, and Bob had been on the list for a month with no heart becoming available. We go to our appointment on Wednesday, and attend the Support group meeting.

It is decided to lower the Melrinone, so new pumps are delivered by Home Health Care that will change the dosage. He will be monitored for changes in heart failure symptoms. Doctors can manage heart failure, but not an infection. If an infection gets into the blood or VAD it could be fatal. Also we went by ICU to visit the nurse he had when he was there, and we ran into one of the ICU doctors; both were happy to see him doing so well.

The next week another appointment with Dermatology, just keep using the cream, can't do much about the rash we are told.

There was a number from his last blood draw that was too low to be on the Transplant List, so our quiet day was another trip for more blood work; you never can tell what a new day will bring.

Second week of September, another follow-up appointment, where we heard they had transplanted a heart this morning. One doctor asked, "Why didn't Washnock get the heart?" It was the wrong blood type, but this indicated he was getting close and when the doctors start talking about it, that is good news. Good check-up, all is going well.

The next morning when Bob woke he was so excited about a dream he had. We watch the "Ellen" show every day; she keeps us laughing, which is just what we need right now, and she does such good things for people. He began to tell me his dream about being on the "Ellen" show and he was telling her about his transplant, the time he spent in the hospital etc. and then she surprised Bob with an English bulldog puppy (he has always wanted one). He was so cute, like a little kid in a candy store. He had a happy day, couldn't stop talking about his dream.

We continue with life, a trip to the storage unit to get a few things, a file for SME (a professional society Bob belongs to). He is working on his SME Auction list, something he has done for many years and will be able to do again. I worked on photo albums, putting the photos on CD's or flash drive.

Bob is showering alone, but I stand by in case he needs help, then we do his dressing change. We are moving along, trying not to think about the Transplant. It will happen when it is his time, and the right one for him comes along.

Saturday night Bob had a dream that he got a call

for his heart and he was speechless in the dream, so he couldn't tell me who was on the phone. Then he woke up; maybe his time is near.

The next week was another appointment, blood draw, chest X-Ray, and a test called a 6-minute walk, a measure of how far he can walk in 6 minutes. They compared the results to one done earlier, and he showed good improvement. Lowering Melrinone again, and will follow him for another couple of weeks, then maybe he can come off this medication. Overall it was a good check-up.

Last week of September and we are still waiting, two months now. Still having Home Health Care come. Bob is up to 1.4 miles on the treadmill, longest walk to date.

Checking out what my friends are doing on Facebook, this week a lot of people we know are in Las Vegas at the Mine Expo. Makes me a little sad that we are home, waiting, and they're out having fun and enjoying life. I know our time will come, and maybe the next Mine Expo we will be able to go.

October is another interesting month with a few bumps in the road. It's Monday and when our Home Care nurse arrived, Bob had an odd look on his face, so she asked him what was happening. Bob said that he just felt a little heart flutter and he was a little light headed, but she checked and his blood pressure and heart rate were fine. She suggested we call the VAD Hot line, so we did, and they want us to send them a report from ICD. We can do that since we have a monitor at home that can transmit information to the hospital. When the hospital called back they asked us to come in for blood work at 1:00 p.m. and clinic at 2:00.

When we arrived we were sent to get an ECHO, and they are trying to figure out if it is V-Tach or suction events from his VAD. These are instances where the VAD may not be getting enough flow. Bob said he feels fine other than that one flutter. It is determined that he had fourteen events on Sunday and nine so far today.

Needless to say, he was admitted to the hospital at 5:30, a right heart cath is scheduled for tomorrow morning, and they are going to keep him for a couple of days to adjust some of his meds; a tune-up so to speak. After a trip home to get Bob his Bi-pap machine and some other things, we watch Monday night football.

Tuesday, continue to monitor Bob, he's doing great. Took him off Melrinone and so far doing well. They will continue to watch him now that he is off, and maybe he can go home tomorrow.

Another person we met in our Support Group meeting was walking around the lobby waiting to be called into surgery; he was told they might have a heart for him today. (He did get his heart, and later we heard was doing well.)

Wednesday, Bob continued to do well, so they are sending us home. Finally arrived home in time for dinner, and a relaxing evening. That night at 3:00 a.m. (now Thursday morning), Bob woke and he said he was nauseous, and had a bad back pain. We tried ginger ale, soda crackers, soda with lemon, but with no change. At 5:00 a.m. we called the VAD Hotline and talked to the nurse on duty; he said to come into the ER to get a CT Scan and see what was happening. What next???

It could be kidney stones, but they are not sure, so Bob is being admitted again. Didn't we just leave?? The plan is to give him antibiotics and watch him to make sure there are no infections, and to do some more tests to find out what it might be.

I went home to shower and get a few things. Most are still packed from yesterday, but in any case, I repack the Bi-Pap machine, IPod, CD player, computer. Who knows how long we will be there this time? What a week!

I returned to the hospital by 1:30 p.m. Bob was getting painkillers, and sleeping most of the time. He tried to eat, but still in a lot of pain, and nauseated. All signs of the heart are good; blood work and flows on the VAD.

Someone from Urology showed up around 6:30 and examined Bob, but couldn't figure out what was causing the pain. No signs of kidney stones on the scan. Maybe he strained a muscle, but a strain would have happened around 10:30 last night, and the upset stomach didn't come until four hours later. Tomorrow another doctor will look at the scan and do another evaluation.

Bob's having trouble peeing. He feels like he needs to, but nothing happens. Is he getting enough water? Just can't figure it out. I decided at go home around 8:00 p.m. I'm so tired; I've been up since 3:00 a.m. Although I tried to nap today, I just couldn't, very worried, praying this doesn't delay a heart if it was Bob's turn.

Friday, Bob is still extremely uncomfortable with stomach pain, no bowel movements and little peeing. Very unusual it seems to me, but the doctors don't seem to be too concerned. Was a long day of pain management, heating pad for his back and muscle relaxants. His back seems better, but the tummy does not. Next plan is to get him something to get his bowels moving. It's possible that all the pain medication could have made him constipated, but the medication would take some time to begin working. I left at 7:30 p.m. Bob was in bed ready to sleep in case he was up all night in the bathroom.

Felt good to get home a little early to relax after another long day at the hospital. Ran into our neighbors Charlie and Debbie, back from Canada for the winter. We talked for a bit and they would like to see Bob and are interested in his progress. Told them Bob could perhaps come home tomorrow, if he had a bowel movement and they figure out this pain.

Saturday, October 6. Still no bowel movement, and extremely tired. The surgeon came in to let us know they had to move Bob to a Status 7 on the Transplant list; he cannot receive a heart, but will continue accumulating time on the list. He explained that Bob is very close to the top of the list and if there is something more going on with his body, they can't transplant until this is resolved.

A decision was made to insert a tube through his nose into his stomach to drain gases and any food. We are told this should help with the bloating but could take until tomorrow.

A quiet sleepy day, napped, passed the time playing games on my tablet with friends most of the day. A sad day, being taken off the active list.

I had a gut feeling that Bob may have missed out on a heart today; just by the way the doctors were talking. I overheard one say it was probably too small anyway, and they discussed Bob's condition and if they should keep him on the list or not. I guess it's not Bob's time. The right one will come along at the right time. Only God knows.

The tube to help the gases isn't working. It's 7:30 p.m. and he is still distended in the stomach and it seems to have gotten worse throughout the day. Another blood draw and then the surgeon came in to tell us he is having a general surgeon see what they can do for Bob. He hasn't peed since yesterday, no poop since Wednesday and today is Saturday. I am so worried as to what is going on. His tummy is pressing on his diaphragm now and causing a shortness of breath. Taking vitals, those all seem to be fine.

Then another heart surgeon came in while they were going to take blood and he said, "No, they can do that downstairs, let's get him moved now!" The general surgeon hasn't arrived yet, but there is talk about maybe having to do surgery to see if there is an obstruction in the bowels.

It's now 8:45 p.m. and Bob is being moved to ICU again. Better to keep an eye on him there. Also putting him back on Melrinone, thinking that taking him off has put a strain on his kidneys. Another PICC line was put in, and an arterial line for pressures was put in. We still don't know what is causing his bloating, but they are going to do more tests, CT Scan, ECHO etc. He must be back on the ventilator to do the ECHO.

The ICU doctor said he hopes that the blood flow to his bowels was not restricted. His breathing has become more labored, and he wants to be on a ventilator to help him breathe. I told him everything will be fine, he is in good hands, and that I was going home to wait. Also I needed to take care of the kitties and pack a few things. Before I left I requested a special nurse for Bob for the next day. He likes her and I think she is Bob's guardian angel in ICU.

It's 1:00 a.m., waiting for a call from the hospital. Dear Lord, I don't know how much more I can take. Finally one of the surgeons called at 1:20. They found what looked like a bowel obstruction but was not. It is called an Ileus, which is a blockage of the intestine (especially the ileum) that prevents the contents of the intestine from passing to the lower bowel. They gave him some meds for it and he is finally passing gas. He should be starting to eliminate very soon, and his bloating is going down, so good news. They are going to do an ECHO next and will call when they get those results tomorrow. He told me that as sick as he looked they were expecting the worst, but it looks better now. They also may be taking the breathing tube out in the next few hours. We will have more details tomorrow.

Thank you Lord. I thought once again that this was the end. This man does have nine lives. I almost left early last night before all this started to happen, but decided to stay. Thank God I did. I thought to myself that if this is heart related, why did they take him off Melrinone? It was working, and why mess up a good thing? I just don't understand, other than it was another area that could get infection.

October 7, Sunday. The nurse called me in the morning; another CT Scan and a PICC line adjustment, since the one last night didn't get in the exact right place being in such a hurry in ICU. He still hasn't had a bowel movement, and also he needs to stay on the ventilator until they are sure they have this figured out, but the bowels are getting blood flow, so it is not as critical as first thought.

When I arrived later in the morning, he was out having his tests. Bob's surgeon came out to talk to me at

11:20 a.m., and told me that Bob was still in his CT Scan, but he does not think it is heart related, as his heart looks the same as last Monday. This may have something to do with his pain and kidneys last Thursday night, when we came into the hospital. They don't know at this point, but he MUST start making urine or they will have to put him on dialysis. I thought to myself, "Oh no, not dialysis too."

A couple of hours later the doctor said, "We think we have it figured out. Bob was fine up until he was given morphine and narcotics for his pain; these drugs can stop a person up. That is why his belly is extended, no bowels movements and no peeing. A colonoscopy is scheduled this afternoon at 3:00 p.m., to take a close look and help clean him out, and hopefully this will get things moving."

An X-Ray of the belly and a cleanout happened at 5:00 p.m., not 3:00 p.m. The procedure took about an hour, and the information I received afterwards was that they did get a lot out and now we just have to wait and see. Keeping him ventilated until they are sure his belly does not bloat up again.

Since Bob is doing a little better and is sedated because of the ventilator, I decided to go home and get a good night's sleep, and also to send an email to all concerned to let them know what had happened the last couple of days. I did call the nurse before I went to bed and he was about the same although his blood pressure was a little low, and he was getting meds for that. Another crazy day!

Monday, October 8, is a total of 128 days in the hospital this year. Last night he was taken off the sedation drugs, so he can be weaned off the ventilator today. He was awake when I arrived, but very sleepy. His fluid retention seems to have gone down a little although his right hand looks a little swollen. It was a long day in ICU.

Urology came by to inform us that he does have a few very small kidney stones and a kidney infection, which is being treated with antibiotics.

Now just wake up so the tube can come out, which it did at 4:30 p.m. A quiet day of sleeping, I napped too. Bob was asking questions and doesn't remember much about the last couple of days.

Back home to sleep, I called before going to bed and he is doing fine, numbers are good and he is sleeping.

Tuesday and Wednesday, a couple more days in ICU. Bob is doing better today. When I talked to him this morning he asked me to bring him some things from home. The doctors said that they are staying the course, he is improving, and his belly is softer. He passed gas this afternoon and is back on clear liquids. A quiet day of rest.

Wednesday started out as a good day, but then he started to complain of a backache that progressively got worse, similar to last Thursday night, same symptoms. May be passing kidney stones, so another Ultrasound will be done to see where they are.

He received pain medication and then slept for a couple of hours, and I managed an hour nap as well. Urination slowed down when he was having pain, but now that the pain is better he is back to normal output. Also able to start back on solid food after a bowel movement; it's the little things that make us happy lately. Who would have thought a bowel movement would make us happy?

Managed to eat a burger, few fries and salad for dinner. After dinner Bob had an emotional moment, and we both began to cry. Bob said, "I am tired of being sick. I just want to be well again," so we hugged and cried together for a while. He can't believe how nice everyone is and how much they care. He thinks so highly of all his doctors.

Thursday and Friday, day 131 in the hospital this year and 12 days this stay. We are back on the Cardiac Floor. This morning Bob showered and dressed, but his back is still hurting, so more medication for pain and a muscle relaxant, being careful not to get too much; we don't want his body stopping up again. He did manage to walk to X-Ray and PT. He must keep strong, he worked so hard all summer to get strong and onto the Transplant list, he can't go backwards.

Then at noon another nosebleed started; it was so bad that the blood backed up and started to come out of his eye socket. It lasted an hour, until ENT made it to the room. They packed the right side this time and took out the packing from the left side. This interfered with his daily PT, and the doctor said he couldn't go home with a nosebleed.

I was not able to go to my Resilience Training class, because Bob wanted me to stay with him; he needs comfort, and likes me there for support. His back continues to hurt, so more painkillers plus heating pad. It seems to be helping but he has had a very tiring day.

Now that we are back on the Cardiac Floor I can start again to bring food from home for Bob's dinner. I have become very creative with meals. When Bob wasn't in ICU, I was microwaving our meals from home in the cafeteria, but then I started using a small crock-pot that I brought, and heated our food in his room. It was okay with the hospital as long as we didn't leave it unattended. This way Bob gets to eat what he likes. After all, hospital food can get very boring after a while.

Arriving home around 9:00 p.m., I found all our clothes in the closet on the floor; the support rods had broken. Just what I needed after the day we had. I moved all the clothes into the other bedroom, all the time cursing and wondering why we have so many clothes. I guess I will buy new supports in the morning. What a day!!! When Bob is miserable, it really tires me out. I get exhausted just watching and being there. Now this happened, more work!

Saturday is a beautiful October day in Arizona. I get my walk in, enjoy a cup of coffee, and a trip to the hardware store for new supports. I began to put some of the clothes away before I return to the hospital, and got dinner ready for tonight.

The plan for the next few days is to wean Bob off Melrinone again, and get his nose under control. A little disagreement between doctors; one wants him to stay on Melrinone and one wants him off to avoid infection, so for now he will come off, but if he has any signs of heart failure he will go back on and stay there until he gets transplanted.

A better day today, less pain, and his nose is consistently weeping from the packing, but not bleeding. We went for a walk to the cafeteria for lunch and then a walk outside; we both managed a nap in the afternoon. Chili for dinner, and then I went home to put more support brackets up and clothes back.

Day 133 this year, and two weeks this stay in the hospital. Was a quiet day of watching football. Bob's nose and eye are very sore from all the bleeding, so he was given a pain medication that helped with his discomfort. Kind of a rough day, so we rested and kept quiet today. The doctor was in and said, "If all goes well, you could go home by Thursday. We want to get you off Melrinone and then do a right heart cath to check your heart function before we send you home." A bit of good news today.

The rest of this week until Thursday was routine, with PT, walks, watching TV, reading etc. Packing came out of his nose on Wednesday, and wept most of the day, but no bleeding. The right heart cath is planned for Thursday morning at 8:00 a.m.; could go home later in the afternoon. As with most procedures it takes longer than expected, also they ran into a blockage from his pacemaker lines, so they had to go through his groin. This makes him need to stay another night, not going home until Friday. Oh well, one more day. We decided that PF Chang's sounded good for dinner since we were not going home.

Friday he was up and dressed; I guess he is ready to go home. We passed the day working on the computer, watching TV, walking, until we finally got word that we are going home. We asked if he will be put back on the Transplant list now, but no, they want to see us in clinic this coming week before they do. We are a little sad, hoping to be back on the list.

It is 137 days in the hospital this year and 19 this stay. What a long year, and it is only October 19. We stop for new prescriptions and takeout pizza for dinner. When we arrived home we were both so tired. There is something about being home that makes a person so relaxed, we are like noodles, veg'ing. Happy to be home together, we will sleep well tonight, or so we thought.

Bob's nose had other plans. Another bleed at midnight, we hold and apply pressure for 20 minutes. No luck, so I called the VAD Hotline for help. Was instructed to pack the nose and hold for twenty minutes; if that didn't work, hold for another ten. Finally by 2:30 a.m. we had the nose under control, and back to sleep.

Saturday through Monday we relaxed, went grocery shopping and really took it easy until we went back for our follow up appointment on Tuesday.

Blood work and doctor appointments, checking Bob out really closely. His blood work looked good, and as of October 23, 2012, he is back on the Transplant List as a 2-B status, the same as he was before this last hospitalization. We are so happy and relieved.

The next week we enjoyed a couple of nights out at friends' house for dinner, grocery shopping, taking walks, just the simple things. The landscapers fixed our sprinkler system, getting things done around the house.

Sunday, October 28. Bob woke with another nosebleed, and this time we couldn't get it to stop and it was a doozy, bleeding everywhere, really scary. Just couldn't get it to slow down, so finally we decided to drive to the hospital. Bob was spitting up blood and blood clots, trying to hold his nose, going through tissues, a towel on his lap, it was crazy. I'm driving as fast and safely as I can to the Emergency Room to get his nose packed.

Two hours later we were on our way home. The packing has to stay in for at least five days. We got home, rested, and watched the World Series and football.

October 29. A day I will never forget. My alarm went off at 6:30 a.m. to get my walk in before Bob gets up. As I was getting out of the bed, Bob's ICD fired, so I called the VAD Hotline, and then it went off again at 6:50, while we were still on the phone. Somehow I managed to get Bob dressed and it fired again. The VAD coordinator told me to call 911. She stayed on the phone with me until the EMT's arrived with ambulances, fire trucks etc.

I was running around watching after the cats, while all these people were coming into my house. They were on the bed putting IV's into Bob, and I was telling them he had a VAD and he couldn't be disconnected from that; they said they knew that.

His ICD kept firing. The EMT was talking to the VAD coordinator at the hospital by this time. EMT's wanted to take Bob to the closest hospital, but the coordinator said NO, he must come to our hospital. We can't, its rush hour and it will take too long to get there. Finally, between them they figured it out to fly him, but from where? The closest hospital? That would take too much time to get him to another hospital then fly him from there, so decided to fly him right from our house.

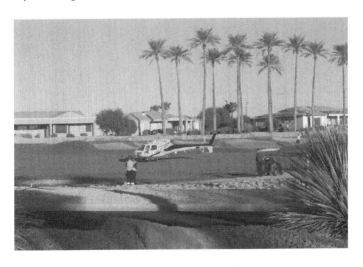

Helicopter waiting to Airlift Bob to the Mayo Hospital

We live at Sun City Grand retirement community and there is a golf course around the corner, so he was loaded into the ambulance and taken to the golf course, where a helicopter was waiting on the 18th hole. I followed them to the helicopter to tell Bob I will be see him at the hospital, I love him, and he will be okay.

The EMT's couldn't believe Bob was awake and talking. His heart was in V-Fib (ventricular fibrillation, a fibrillation of the heart muscles resulting in interference with rhythmic contractions of the ventricles and possibly leading to cardiac arrest), but in Bob's case his LVAD kept the blood flowing throughout his body and kept him alive.

I drove through rush hour and made it in fifty minutes, whereas Bob made it in eight minutes in the helicopter. When he arrived in the ER, a magnet was placed onto his pacemaker to stop it from firing. It's like getting kicked in the chest by a mule. His ICD fired twenty-three times in ninety minutes; that is a lot of getting hit in the chest. All of his doctors, I think there were five of them, the VAD coordinator, plus other staff from ER were all standing by.

When I arrived, he was resting with a little sedation, but still awake enough to know I was there. Now it's time to figure out what happened! Why didn't his ICD bring him out of this V-Fib? Why did it keep firing? These are questions that have to be answered.

Once Bob was stable he was moved to ICU, where he slept most of the day. Getting shocked that many times really took a toll on him. I went home to shower and get a few things once again, preparing for another stay in the hospital. Upon returning, Bob was sleeping and they are going to let the heart rest for a couple of days before putting it through more shock, which is what needs to be done to test the ICD to find out what happened.

Tuesday, October 30, 139 days this year and 21 days this month. Bob is moved up on the Transplant List to 1-A status (highest on the list) for the next twenty-eight days. If a heart does not come during that time frame, and he goes home, he will be lowered to a 1-B status. As long as he stays in the hospital he will remain 1-A on the list. When the twenty-eight days ends, they can petition to remain 1-A status on a weekly basis, providing he is in the hospital and his condition remains the same.

EP was in, changed his pacemaker to 80 bpm (beats per minute); this may help him sleep better. It was at 100 bpm, which they seemed to think was a little fast. Another day of resting and waiting, so with Bob being fairly stable today, I went home to make dinner for tomorrow as I do every night.

Wednesday, October 31st, Halloween. Was a quiet day for Bob, no events, and he was moved to the Cardiac Floor, where he was able to shower and take a few short walks.

Had a visit from another Transplant patient we met earlier in the year, and he is doing well. We were talking about another patient we got to know quite well last winter; he had passed away. It was so sad - he had struggled for many months with poor lung capacity and kidney function, and just couldn't get strong enough to get on the Transplant list. We got to know his wife and father while we were both in and out of ICU; we were good support for each other for many months. He finally had enough and did not want to be put on life support any longer, and his family granted his wishes. He was only in his forties. We are so grateful that Bob has no other major issues to keep him from getting on the list. Our hearts go out to his family.

We are excited and scared waiting for a heart, being so close to the top of the list. Don't know how I will feel when word comes that they have a match. There are always risks, life or death. It's hard to imagine what that feeling will be like and how to express it. Will it be jubilation? Nervous? Scared? Or will we be numb and in shock? Only time will tell.

Thursday, November 1. We are told we will be staying in the hospital at least for the weekend, in hopes of a donor heart. Also, his ICD needs to be tested before we can go home. We found out that they had an offer for a heart for Bob when he was having his kidney stones and belly problems a couple of weeks ago. It just wasn't meant to be. God had his plan.

On one of our walks to the gift shop today we ran into a couple of the Transplant coordinators, and they called Bob a saint for all he has been through. They also said that the entire team will be jubilant when he finally gets his heart. Bob is so well liked and that is good to hear, and why not, he is a wonderful man.

My friend Judy came by for a visit - always good to see her. She brought her usual glass of wine, one for her and one for me.

The weekend was spent walking, watching TV, trying to keep busy and not think about the heart. Having a good day, we walked to the cafeteria for lunch. When we got back to the room and were doing puzzles, his nose started to bleed. Again the ENT's came and packed his nose, so it's time to rest.

Sunday had a visit from our neighbors Charlie and Debbie, walked, napped, and moved to a larger corner room, with a table, chairs, and a couch.

I was thinking today how few friends we had come to visit, and usually the same ones. Makes you wonder who really cares or not, and who your real friends are. We have each other and that is what really matters. I know it is a drive to get to the hospital, but a friend would take the time, like Judy. Her drive is forty-five minutes, and she comes a couple times a week. We did have some friends that came from Tucson, but local people not so much.

One of the doctors paid a visit and said to keep quiet, meaning his heart. He also informed us that they have to test Bob's ICD before going home to make sure it is working properly, and when they get tired of us they will send us home. Funny!! Tasty dinner from PF Chang's.

The next week was more waiting, working out in the gym on strengthening, walking outside, keeping busy, TV, puzzles, internet games, reading, going to the support group meetings, etc. Looks like they want to keep Bob here until his twenty-eight days are up, in hopes a donor becomes available.

Finally got the packing out of his nose on Thursday, and Friday was the one-year anniversary of being put on the TP list the first time, although he was on and off this past year.

We were walking and holding hands one day and one of Bob's doctors saw us and said, "Cutest couple in the hospital, walking and holding hands. Keep up the good work!"

Another weekend is upon us, watching more football, walking, and waiting. His heart has been quiet and steady since the helicopter ride. That's good news.

On Monday Bob woke to yet another, can you believe it, nosebleed, so it was packed again. Something needs to be done. The ENT doctor recommended ligation to stop the blood flow to the nose. Two doctors agreed and one did not. The Transplant surgeon was concerned about him being on life support and a nosebleed starting. "I can't stop a heart transplant to deal with a nosebleed," one of them said. It was decided to do the procedure tomorrow, a small surgery to cut the vessels causing the bleeds; should take a couple of hours. NPO (nothing by mouth) after midnight. When they may not be able to do the surgery until the afternoon, it's a very long day of waiting, unless we get a heart tonight or they can do the procedure in the morning. We will see what happens tomorrow.

Tuesday, lucky day, he was taken at 11:00 a.m. for the procedure, but then waited in pre-op until 2:00 p.m., not so lucky. Then the doctor came in and said there were a couple of emergency Cardiac surgeries going on and the Cardiac anesthesiologists were all busy, so we can wait and have it later tonight or wait until Thursday morning. Bob opted to wait until Thursday so that he could eat; he was so hungry.

Just hanging out this Wednesday, waiting for his procedure tomorrow, again NPO after midnight. This time he was taken at 6:30 a.m.; the doctor called me at 9:40 and said that he did really well, and was in recovery. I was waiting in his room when he arrived back at 12:20. Light lunch of PB&J, slept most of the afternoon, really woke up around 5:00 in time for dinner. Overall a good day and a fix for the nosebleeds, we hope.

A quiet weekend, although Bob is complaining

about not going to the bathroom, very constipated and concerned. His nose is oozy as well. Finally decided to have the nurse give him an enema.

Sunday, our neighbor John came by to watch football so I went out shopping for a wedding shower gift, and ran into a couple of other stores. I found a great crock-pot that has three sections that I thought would be perfect for Thanksgiving dinner. It felt good to get out and have some "retail therapy" time. It's been 158 days this year in the hospital and 24 this time around.

Thanksgiving week didn't start out so good. Bob woke to a nosebleed at 4:30 a.m. and when I arrived he was sitting on the edge of the bed, crying and upset. It's 11:15 and the ENT doc is trying to get him into the clinic and ablate his nose again, but no luck. It's not something they can do in clinic. His nose bleeds because of his blood thinners, which he needs because he is on the LVAD. The only thing that could stop this is a new heart and to get off blood thinners. Not much else can be done at this time other than pack his nose again, which they do. Needless to say, it was a quiet day of rest after the events of this morning. We had dinner and then I left early to get groceries for Thanksgiving dinner.

Wednesday, my friend Candy arrived again from Chile, pre-wedding, and we get take-out for dinner for the three of us, then she and I go home to prepare Thanksgiving dinner to bring to the hospital tomorrow. So fun to be with my best friend for a few hours, sharing all the Thanksgiving dinner prep, drinking wine, laughing, a little crying and really having a fun night.

Thanksgiving morning we woke early to get the turkey

in the oven and prepare all the side dishes and pumpkin pie. Packed all the food in containers, loaded the car with coolers of food, crock pots to warm dinner, tablecloths, cloth napkins, dishes and silverware.

We did get sidetracked and ended up going to a few golf shops in the area, but made it to the hospital by 2:00 p.m. in time to unload and began warming up our Thanksgiving dinner. I suppose we were quite a sight as we borrowed a cart and loaded it with all this crockery and containers and wheeled it through the lobby and up the elevator and into Bob's room.

We set up our "fancy" Thanksgiving dinner table and watched football while our dinner was warming, and ate around 4:00. Dinner turned out just great, so tasty, even with it being warmed over. Candy's son David came by and also her daughter Gretchen with her fiancée Logan. Really had a nice Thanksgiving Day. Candy left with her children around 7:00; I changed Bob's dressing and then went home, finished cleaning, doing dishes and putting food away. Even though we spent the holiday in the hospital we made the best of it and had a good day.

Friday when I arrived they were taking the packing out of Bob's nose, and somehow it had moved to the back of his throat and it came out through his mouth, yucky and gross. It was suggested that he keep a cotton ball with Vaseline on it inside his nostrils to prevent it from drying out. It's better than packing, and if it works, that will be great.

Our neighbor Denise came for a visit, and the two of us went out for lunch; her husband John stayed at home as he was not feeling very good and didn't want to share any germs with Bob.

We had take-out Mexican food for dinner, which seems to be our usual Friday night dinner lately. Stayed until 8:00 and drove home.

We had a quiet weekend. I bought a HDMI cable so Bob could get the football games on his laptop that he can't get on TV. Our other neighbors, Charlie and Deb, arrived for a visit around 5:00 and we decided to order pizza. Yes, they deliver pizza to the hospital. Sounds odd, but as long as Bob stays within his sodium count for the day, at this point he can eat almost anything. We had a nice visit, they left around 7:00 and I got home around 8:45 p.m., getting dinner ready for tomorrow.

One of the doctors came by earlier in the day, but I missed him. Bob said he didn't have much to say other than Bob's heart is on back order. For him we thought that was kind of funny, since he is usually all business. It's nice to see a sense of humor.

The next couple of days of waiting, we are told they haven't even had any offers for hearts come in, so it's been quiet on that account. Planning on testing Bob's ICD tomorrow to make sure it is working properly, in order to send him home as a 2-B status.

He only has a day and a half left on his 1-A status. If his ICD is not working properly, they can't send him home unless they replace it, and they really don't want to have Bob go through another surgery. If it is not working, they will keep him in the hospital until a donor heart is a match.

Next day, he goes through the testing during which they increase his heart rate so high as to make the ICD fire the heart into beating normally. If it works, great, we go home. Well, it didn't take him out of his arrhythmia; they actually had to use the paddles manually four times to get his heart out of the arrhythmia.

When he arrived back to his room he was still a little sedated, and he had burn marks on his upper body where they used the paddles to shock his heart. He was sore and tired. We used a burn balm on the marks, but they took a week to heal.

Based on the testing, they decided to keep Bob in the hospital until a donor heart was available, and they would petition the donor organization to keep him as a 1-A status. We don't know if we are happy or not - staying in the hospital waiting, or going home and worrying about his ICD firing. We decided that the best place for Bob is in the hospital, and once we made peace with that decision, we were fine to wait.

Little did we know we would be there for a few more *MONTHS*, but during that time we made the best of our stay. The following is what we did in the time we waited, not so much a day to day journal but our life as we knew it then, another new normal.

Chapter 4

Waiting For A Donor Heart

November 28, 2012, our next phase of the journey begins. 168 days in the hospital this year and 33 days this stay. Gretchen's wedding is this weekend. On Thursday, I went out for dinner with friends that are in town for the wedding and stayed overnight with Candy at her hotel. We had a wonderful time reminiscing and wishing Bob was there with us.

Friday was the wedding shower and a lovely luncheon. Bob called Gretchen and told her that wild horses couldn't keep him away from her wedding, but apparently the Cardiac doctors could. She cried - Gretchen has known us all of her life, and wanted him at her wedding, but it was not to be.

As for myself, I was so torn. I wanted Bob to go, but was truly afraid that he would have an episode, and need sudden emergency treatment, and ruin the event for the bride.

Saturday, the wedding day. I arrived at the hospital and spent most of the day with Bob, then got ready for the wedding in his room. One of my friends had this great idea to "Skype" the wedding to Bob in the hospital. We called Bob and he was able to find a phone to watch the ceremony live. I also had my tablet and recorded the ceremony on that. It was such a beautiful event and reception. The only one missing was my sweetheart Bob. Later that night the girls got together after the reception and had a little wine and talked way into the night; we had such fun.

Some friends that were in town to attend the wedding came to visit Bob at the hospital the next day. A woman from our support group that was transplanted stopped for a visit, too. The doctors also asked Bob to talk to a patient that is considering an LVAD. We visited with her for a while and she was having some of the same feelings and reservations that Bob had and has - not feeling well, no appetite, scared. I think Bob put her at ease.

We attend the weekly support group meetings, PT and Cardiac Rehab continue, also recreational therapy, where we go daily to bowl on the Wii, we also takes walks outside.

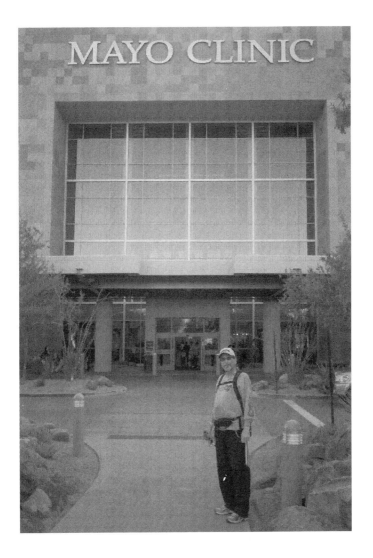

Walking Outside of the Mayo

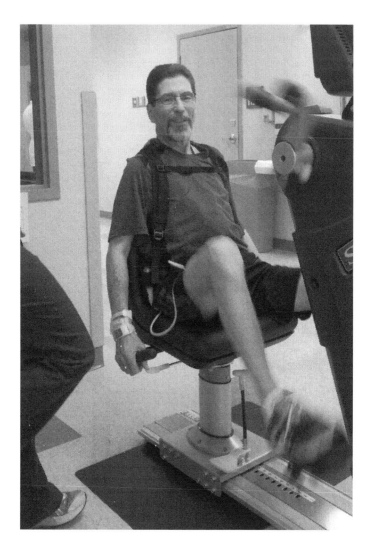

Exercising Waiting For Transplant

December 10, Bob has another nosebleed and it must be packed again; so sad. The oblation surgery didn't work; his blood is just thin. Doctors are hopeful a heart will come before the end of the year.

A beautiful day, December 13th - my birthday. I had a fun birthday lunch at an outside patio setting, with girlfriends Candy, Judy, and newlywed Gretchen.

Busy week bringing Christmas decorations into Bob's room - a small table tree, bulbs, lights, wreath, and garland. Sure makes his room cheery and everyone comments on how nice it looks. Candy brought over some heart ornaments – so cute. She told the story that while shopping for them in a local craft store, she was told that hearts are normally available only in February, not December, but when she explained why she was looking for them (for her friend on the heart transplant list) before she knew it, two customers and a clerk were helping her scour the store for something she could use to create them. It is so nice to experience such kindness from strangers.

I continue to bring in homemade dinners and lunch from time to time. Nurses are looking into our room at dinnertime to see what's on the menu. They say it always smells so good that they have to come and see what's cooking.

The week before Christmas I'm busy making Christmas cookies and peanut brittle in the evenings when I get home from the hospital, and on those nights I leave early. I tell Bob that if he wants cookies, I must get home, and he agrees. Also busy doing a little Christmas shopping for Bob and since Bob can't get out and shop, I shop for myself and wrap them as if he bought them for me. Also getting packages mailed to family. If he gets a heart and is home for Christmas, great, but if not, we are prepared to celebrate in the hospital, and make it a joyous holiday day.

Bob was again asked to talk to another patient in ICU waiting for an LVAD. He is really sick and needs this operation, although he is not sure if he wants it. After talking to Bob, he felt much better about the device.

December 23rd. I did my grocery shopping for the holiday dinners - Shish-ka-bobs for Christmas Eve, and steak, lobster, baked potato and Caesar salad for Christmas day. Christmas Eve we watched Scrooge then I went home to prepare Christmas dinner.

December 25th, 196 days in the hospital this year and Day 62 this stay. We never would have thought back in October we would be here for Christmas. Here it is Christmas morning, getting up at 6:00 a.m. to arrive early at the hospital, so we could go to the cafeteria for breakfast and have omelets, which is what we usually have at home on Christmas morning. Later that morning we opened gifts. I made a Mimosa for myself, like I would have at home, and Bob had juice. Watched a couple of Christmas movies, "Polar Express" and "Santa Claus" in the afternoon. We enjoyed a nice dinner with linens and Christmas dishes I brought from home. So overall we made the best of the holiday, just the two of us.

The rest of this year 2012, we kept as busy as one can, being in the hospital. Friends in town for the holidays would come and visit, and were happy to see Bob doing so well.

Before I left the house on New Year's Eve morning, I had to cover the plants, since it is going to freeze tonight (a rarity). I also decided to stay close to the hospital, so I wouldn't have to drive with all the crazies on the road, in case we get the call for a heart.

New Year's Eve day we are talking to the nurses and doctors, wishing them a Happy New Year, when Bob says, "It would be nice to have a glass of champagne to toast the New Year," so the Transplant coordinator asked his doctor and he said yes, just one small glass. So off I go to the wine store to buy a nice bottle of champagne. When I got there they were having a tasting and I was able to taste a few champagnes, and decided on Tesoro Della Regina, which turned out to be very good. Also stopped to buy a couple of champagne glasses since home was 45 minutes away and you can't drink champagne out of paper cups!

We ordered takeout from PF Chang's for dinner. We had a nice quiet New Year's Eve, made a toast and celebrated early, since I was tired and wanted to get settled in my room. We both watched the ball drop but in separate places. Overall our evening was about the same as it would have been at home, other than being apart at midnight. Happy New Year 2013! Let's pray it's a good one.

Arrived at the hospital at 9:00 a.m., so that Bob and I could go to the cafeteria for our traditional New Year's breakfast, omelets, toast and juice. Had a nice quiet holiday watching football most of the day and a nap here and there. I had prepared dinner the day before at home, which was shrimp cocktail, caesar salad, filet, and a baked potato. One of doctors was in and said, "This is the year." Well, it wasn't last year and I sure as heck hope we don't have to wait until next year. We laughed.

January 4, 2013. It is one year since he had his LVAD

surgery. Wow, where has the time gone? We never thought a year ago that we would still be in this situation, but we are and we are doing fine.

Our neighborhood is busy taking down the Christmas lights. My neighbor John had taken down ours one day while I was at the hospital - such a great guy. Then I finished taking the lights off the palm trees, and got all the decorations put away and organized in the garage. I noticed the golf cart is not charging, so I deal with that, but it looks like we will need new batteries. I think that can wait for a while.

We received news that there may have been a heart for Bob, but something about it just wasn't right, so the doctors turned it down. They are very particular. The only thing is, we wish we hadn't heard about it. Kind of a letdown feeling, so close. But the time just isn't right, and when the right one comes along it will be a good one.

The month of January 2013, another month of waiting, feeling frustrated at times. It's one thing to be in the hospital and not feeling well and another to be feeling pretty good and there is nothing anyone can do to get a heart, only God knows. We must be patient for the right one to come along. We continue our life at the hospital, trying to keep busy. This is now our new normal for the time being. Friends come to visit; we go for walks outside for fresh air, eat, sleep and survive.

On Martin Luther King Day they had a tape playing in one of the conference rooms, and since neither of us had heard his entire speech, we thought we would go and listen. We did and it was inspiring. We do things like this to keep us occupied.

Bob works on his auction for the SME conference in February; this keeps him busy part of his day. Patients come and go, weather changes, life goes on. I continue my walks and preparing food to take with me daily.

There are times when I am so tired of the same thing, the driving back and forth every day, preparing food and packing it up. I have my good days and bad. I have a good cry and I'm okay for a while, but it is very frustrating, my neck hurts from the stress and I am just plain tired. Neighbors I run into ask about Bob, seems like daily; everyone is praying for him.

February 2013, starts out the same other than we were having a burger and fries for lunch one day, and one of his doctors came in and didn't seem very happy about his choice of food. Said, "Enjoy it now because after transplant it's low fat and heart healthy diet," which we are aware of and will follow as closely as we can. We didn't let it bother us; we still have to live and enjoy life.

Valentine's Day, I stop and buy Valentine balloons and a card for Bob. We are hoping this will be the day - wouldn't it be nice to get a new heart on Valentine's Day? But no luck today.

We had a little spat. Bob wanted this new cologne and I said that he seems to have enough and should use what he has first. Then he snapped at me and said, "You buy what you want, but when I ask for something it's always, 'do you need it?' or question what I want." It made me feel really bad and I cried. He apologized and said that he was sorry, that he was a little touchy and on edge with all this waiting. We hugged, kissed and everything was okay.

Although when I got home I had another good cry.

Why is this happening to us and how long do we have to wait? What did we do to deserve this? I just needed to let off some steam. Had a couple of glasses of wine and cried myself to sleep.

One day I was cutting Bob's hair and the doc came in. He just smiled and said to be careful, he is on blood thinners; it was funny and we enjoyed it. We would sit on the patio and do puzzles, reading the paper or books on nice days.

Chapter 5

The New Heart

February 19th, 2013. My usual morning, cup of coffee, then was getting ready for my walk around 8:00 a.m., and the phone rang. It was Bob and he said, "There is a possibility of a heart today. They NOP'd me," (that's nothing by mouth). I was so excited; my heart began to pound, nervous and excited, yet scared all at the same time. I always wondered how I would feel. There you have it - a bag full of mixed emotions. So I immediately showered and got ready to spend a few nights at the hospital or near it.

When I arrived around 10:00 a.m. there was no news yet, so Bob showered, we walked and tried to keep our minds busy; this could take hours to happen. On our walk we talked, and Bob told me that I have taught him what unconditional love is, by taking care of him, bringing food from home, and just being there every day, never missing one day in 274 days in the hospital, since this ordeal started back in 2011. We cried and made plans and just talked about if anything should happen to him and what to do. We love each other so much; God wouldn't take him from me now.

When we returned from our walk, we were told it was a no-go; there were two others ahead of him and one of them got the heart. What a downer this news was. A while later the doctor came to our room and we asked him the reason. He said, "Bob was 3rd in line and now he is 2nd." Another doctor poked his head in and said, "We came close." Bob thought that was nice of him to do that. So now that Bob can eat, he had a little snack to hold him over until dinner. After all the excitement we both took a nap. Then I picked up take-out from PF Chang's for dinner, watched TV and I went home. What a day!!

Oops, it's not over. Bob called me at 10:33 p.m. and asked if I was sleeping. No, I was just getting into bed. He said, "You know they said it would happen when you least expect it, well they are prepping me for surgery, blood draws, IV's etc." Wow, here we go again!

I am on my way. Made it back in an hour after Bob called. They are washing his body. A couple of nurses came in and began shaving him from the groin to the chin. Changed him into a gown, took him to pre-op (I was able to go with him too), where they continued to get him ready. The Profusionist was there to take care of his LVAD. It is now 1:00 a.m. and we are waiting for the rest of the surgical team and anesthesiologist.

2:15 a.m. The surgeon came in to see us and said that there is always a chance it might not go. They have to make sure the heart is good and good for Bob. In the meantime there was a PA changing doctors' appointments for the morning since they would be in surgery, having a hard time reaching other patients. It was a very busy time for everyone. We said our "see you later" hugs and kisses. I'm crying. Bob talked about if he didn't make it, he wanted to be cremated and his ashes spread over Mt. Ripley in the Upper Peninsula of Michigan. I could make other arrangements, and he wanted a memorial service as well. Off to surgery at 2:20 a.m. the morning of February 20, 2013, with two of the best Cardiothoracic surgeons in the world. What a great team he has.

I went back to pack his room and load it in the car, feeling drained. He sure had accumulated a lot of stuff in that little room. It was raining. The Head Floor nurse said I could stay in his room until shift change at 7:00 and try to get a little sleep. Surprisingly, I managed to do that for a few hours. I left his room at shift change, got a little breakfast, and then checked into the waiting room. One of the nurses that we know really well came to see me and said she had heard that they didn't open him up until 5:00 a.m., so I wait. It could be many hours yet. It's a cold and rainy day; glad to be inside.

At 8:15 a.m. another nurse came to see how I was doing, and said it will be a while yet. She was heading to ICU to let some of the others know about Bob. Just sitting around, I called my sister, Bob's son Derek, his brother, and my friends Candy and Judy. Playing games online with Candy to help pass the time. I have no idea who won or even what we played.

11:30 a.m. I decided I needed a walk. While I was out walking the waiting room called and said the doctor called from surgery and said, "Tell Mrs. Washnock her husband now has a new heart as of 11:46 a.m.!" WOW!! I cried, called my sister and Candy, sent a quick email to family and will update the rest when I have more info. Went back to the waiting room for the doctors to come and talk to me.

Finally at 3:00 p.m. the doctors appeared, and they were smiling. They said, "All went well and he has a GOOD heart. He will be in his room in ICU in about half an hour and you can see him then." I was so relieved!!!

I went to grab a bite to eat, and ran into one of his nurses in the lobby; she gave me a big hug and was so happy for the good news.

Soon I was able to go and see Bob; he is on a ventilator but resting, his numbers look good, and he is being constantly monitored. His blood pressure began to drop and meds were adjusted, which helped bring it back to where they want it. The heart transplant coordinators, nurses, doctors, PA's, and so many of the staff keep coming by to see us. Such a wonderful feeling to have all this support and knowing they all care so much and are so happy for us. I hung out until after rush hour, knowing he would be sedated the rest of the night, and he is in good hands.

Neighbors stopped by while I was unloading the car. John and Denise happened to be coming home, and ran over to give me hugs, so excited. John said, "Everyone has been praying for you," and told me that he admires me for being there every day and cooking - he even told his church about us. We had lots of good wishes and prayers all day.

I poured a glass of wine, and called to check on Bob. His nurse said he was stable and starting to respond to commands like wiggle toes and hands. Thank you thank you, dear God. Good night.

Day 1 of New Heart

I had a good night's sleep, got ready, so excited and joyful this morning - it's going to be a good day. I called Bob's nurse before I left the house. His nurse said Bob is doing great; the plan is to lower the Nitric Oxide and the ventilator support. Bob is breathing on his own and needing very little help from the machines.

I arrived and cried from happiness - he was somewhat awake and motioned with his hands "I Heart You." Then he motioned to parts of his body where his ICD and LVAD were, asking if they were gone, and I told him that all his extra hardware is gone, just a new heart. He looks relieved and tries to smile, but he can't yet. He has to wait a few more hours before they can take out his vent tube.

Lots of staff is stopping by to congratulate Bob. The transplant coordinators stopped by and said that the heart was the same one offered yesterday morning, but that the other recipient decided not to take it; we don't know why. What a miracle!

Judy and I went for lunch to celebrate and when I returned he was off the ventilator. We had a quiet and restful day, since he is still very sleepy. Having some pain later in the day but they gave him medication for it. I left around 7:00 p.m.

Day 2 New Heart

Well, what a night. I went to bed early thinking I needed a good night's sleep, but I had trouble getting to sleep and was still awake at 10:30 p.m. Woke at 5 a.m., and couldn't get back to sleep. Guess I'm thinking everything is going so well and Bob is doing so well, but yet I am waiting for something bad to happen. Anyway, I get up, have coffee and text and play games until it's light out, then I go for my morning walk.

Arrive at the hospital around 10:30, and Bob is doing well. Nurses, PT, and more are stopping by to say hi and congratulations; everyone is so happy for Bob. Doctors informed us he could eat solid food, so we split a burger and each had a salad. I left around 7:30, tired. I am sure it will take a few days to get rested up after all the excitement and lack of sleep the last few nights.

It's now day 3 for his new heart

54 days this year in the hospital, 120 days since the helicopter brought him in last October, and a total of 277 days since this all began in 2011. I slept in and ran a few errands, arriving around 11:00 a.m. Bob was sitting up in the chair and also had his first walk this morning. His external pacemaker was turned off. It had been helping his new heart work, not unusual after a transplant. He is taking his meds by mouth, off IV's except Dobutamine, and some fluids.

Bob is not real happy about his diet restrictions - Cardiac Diet, Diabetic Diet, low sodium and fluid restrictions. Besides not liking the hospital food, he is having a hard time finding anything to eat that he likes. When he is moved to the cardiac floor I will be able to bring food from home. He was a picky eater before his new heart, and he remains picky, no surprise there.

Napping in the afternoon, he must have been dreaming and began to talk in his sleep. He barked at one point, "He was going to buy a tile kit…I don't know how much those bags are, $125 bucks? They are coming at 1:00, what are we going to do with them? Some of those guys have pretty big bellies on them, don't they?" Just dreaming strange things. He said, "Donna," then his lips looked like he was kissing, go figure, then he settled down. It's amazing what drugs can do to a person, he was sedated for so long in surgery it's no wonder he is having strange dreams. We ate dinner, and then I left to go home.

The Following Days

The next day one of his doctors said that all this talk could be caused by the medication Prednisone he is on. He is still dreaming and talking in his sleep again today. Some of what he was saying, "He hit it out of the ball park and they didn't call it a home run. I see all these kids bringing all this stuff to school." I asked him if he was dreaming and he said, "Yes." He knew that I had come in, and he gave me a kiss. Still talking, "I'm injured. What's he doing?" "That's a pretty good size Cuban. Hey what do you know sir? White sauce with pino? Four kinds of bread and toast you take before they pull the tubes," plus talking about marinating chicken - just crazy talk.

We were excited that the chest tubes that drain excess fluid were coming out, but then they found a little fluid in his right lung, so they are waiting another day. Evening nurses will take out the catheter and get Bob cleaned up tonight, so I decided to go home.

Now I can't quite explain, except to say that it has been a couple of trying days for me, but when I got home I started to cry. I just want to see Bob normal again. Seeing him mumble and talk nonsense is hard. I never expected it, and it really drains my energy. As the steroids are lowered it will get better and I have to remind myself of this. We have come so far; we can make it through this too. For those of you reading this, remember that this is a long journey. You may think that we have a new heart, so now everything is going to be back to normal and just fine. It isn't. It takes time and patience.

Arriving the next morning, I find the wound care nurses checking out Bob's bedsores on his feet, bum, and head. The feet are looking better, the bum is slightly red, and his head is losing hair from where the sore is, but overall they said they were looking better.

The chest tubes come out in the morning and after lunch the IV from the neck came out and they put a new one in his arm. Moving out of ICU this afternoon as soon as a room is ready on the cardiac floor. While we wait we nap, and Bob continues to talk in his sleep.

We finally make it to the cardiac floor at 4:00. Before he left ICU he was given Lasix for fluid retention, something for his blood pressure and they took him off Dobutamine. Usually they wean off slowly but they didn't this time. While in transport Bob was fine, but when they hooked him up to the monitors on the floor, his heart rate and blood pressure were lower than they like. So the heart failure team said to give him more fluids, put him back on the external pacemaker and see what happens.

The surgeon came in, took over, and adjusted the pacemaker for the right side of the heart and his pressure and heart rate came back to where they want it. Heart rate and pressures need to be in a certain range for a new heart, and the doctor got it back there.

Bob slept for a couple of hours and seemed more awake after his nap. He sat in a chair for dinner, chili from home, and he ate pretty good, then back to bed. The evening nurse said, "It's time for you to begin to ask for your meds, so you ring me at 8:00 p.m. and again at 8:00 a.m. You need to start remembering when you need to take your meds and what meds you are getting, so let's start now."

This is good, because we will have to remember when we get home. I told the nurse that he is so out of it, and about the weird side effects from the meds and that she should check on him, and she said, "Of course we will, we wouldn't let him forget."

So the way the doctors are assigned is, the surgeons are the main doctors until they move to the cardiac floor, then the heart failure team takes over. Sometimes a Fellow will check in and it seems to me that they don't always know what is going on. Like a question the Fellow asked was, "Why is Bob so tired?" I told him it's because he doesn't sleep at night from the steroids, so he sleeps during the day. I would think he should know that, but then again maybe not. The surgeons seem to be more aggressive and act faster than the other team. I like faster, not "let's wait and see." I feel more assured that they know what they are doing.

The surgeon could tell I was a little upset about the Fellow's ignorance and assured me that Bob is fine and we just want the numbers where a new heart should be. I think I need to talk to the doctors in charge tomorrow to get this clear in my mind.

The last few days with Bob not sleeping and talking crazy have really taken a toll on me; I am tired and frustrated. I know this will pass but for now it's what I have to deal with, and it's hard. They don't prepare you for this because everyone is different, but I think they should tell you what could happen and help prepare the loved ones.

The sixth day after transplant, I finally had a good night's sleep, went for my morning walk and off to the hospital. When I arrived, Bob was getting ready for a walk. He did take a good walk and looks 100% better today than yesterday. The surgeon was in checking on his pacemaker and made an adjustment. He said that his heart is doing all the work, and if it falls below a certain threshold the pacemaker will kick in, but right now the new heart is working good. This made me feel better after yesterday, knowing he is on top of it.

Bob is more awake today. He had a chest x-ray, lunch, and napped. His friend Errol came in for a visit; good to see him and he was happy Bob was doing so well.

Bob realized he had to poop; the nurse gave him an enema, and he finally had a BM after a week. He was worried about not having one, so this eased his mind. We didn't want to have another bump in the road to recovery.

Then the nurse noticed Bob's right arm was a little swollen. They took out the IV, and called for a PICC nurse to put in a new one. We napped and he was dreaming crazy dreams again. He asked me, "Who was beating his girlfriend? Was it Harry?" I said, "No, you are dreaming," then he said, "What's in the way, pipe or wires?" Just nuts!

A much better day all around. I feel better to realize that Bob is coming back and more awake today. I went home to make beef barley soup for tomorrow night's dinner.

Day 7, another busy day. When I arrived, the PICC nurse was putting in another IV, since the one from last night was hurting him. The Cardiac Team, about six of them, was in doing their rounds. They just told us the plan for the next couple of days is to do another ECHO and a biopsy. This is called endomyocardial biopsy, where the physician takes a tiny piece of tissue from the heart and examines it under a microscope to look for signs of rejection. The biopsy takes about thirty minutes and is done under local anesthesia. Rejection is when the immune system has been "turned on" and is actively defending the body against the transplanted organ. Rejection may occur at any time after transplant, but most often occurs within the first few weeks to months after. However, rejection does not mean that your heart is going to fail. Rejection is expected and may be managed by changing the dosage of immunosuppressant medications.

We had lunch and went to the Transplant Meeting. The couple from California was here, going through the evaluation process to see if he was eligible for a heart transplant. While he was going through the process, the doctors admitted him into the hospital. His heart was so bad that he needed to be monitored and put on IV medication. He and his wife were both extremely upset. He looked scared and she couldn't stop crying - I sure know how they feel. You know when people say you don't know what it's like? Well, we can say for certain we *do* know, and so we talked to them and gave them encouragement. He didn't know if he wanted to have a transplant or not, but really, what other option is there?

After the meeting, I ran into his wife crying in the lobby, so we talked and I tried to encourage her, as best as I could. I told her that in the beginning I cried all the time, and when I didn't think I had another tear to shed, it started all over. I told her that finally one day driving to the hospital it occurred to me that I was scared, scared of the unknown, and that's why I cried so much, and once I figured it out, the tears were still there on some days, but at least I knew why.

Later that day we ran into both of them again. He told us after seeing Bob a week after Transplant and how well he was doing, that he made the decision to go ahead and have the transplant. We were so happy that he made the right decision, and it was all because we went to the meeting and they were there.

Later in the afternoon, Bob had his ECHO and then went for his biopsy. The ECHO came back great; his ejection fraction was at 71%, but they couldn't do the biopsy in the neck. They found a blockage in his neck where they wanted to go to get to the heart for the biopsy. The doctor explained that it was because he had an ICD and lines running from the right side, so he had a lot of scar tissue built up. They couldn't go through the left side because his anatomy wouldn't allow it, so we will have to do his biopsies from the groin, and it will be tomorrow.

So we had dinner, Judy came for a visit, and I went home to start cleaning the house and getting ready to bring Bob home, whenever that would be.

Thursday is day 8 after transplant. A biopsy in the morning, so he is sleepy and groggy from the drugs most of the day. Napping a lot, this is fine since he must lie still for four hours after the procedure. PT got him up and walking later in the day.

Although his arm is still swollen, no one from the heart failure team seemed to be too concerned. One of Bob's surgeons who had been out of town for a few days came by and said, "Heard good things about you, that you are doing well." We asked him about his arm, and he said he will call the heart failure team, and they got right on it. Soon they had his arm elevated and it is slowly getting better. An ultrasound was ordered to check his right arm and why it may be swollen.

The rest of the afternoon was nurses attending to his dressings, wound care nurse checking on his bed sores, nutrition coming by with information on a 2400 calorie a day diet, low sodium but not low fat, diabetic diet as well; more education to take home with us.

Resting and waiting for ultrasound. They arrived around 6:45 p.m. to check on your neck to see what is going on with the right arm. Received news at 8:00 p.m. that he has a blood clot, which means blood thinners until it is dissolved. It is in an area where it would not travel due to the scar tissue and blockage in his neck, so good news, but bad news we will have to stay in hospital for a few more days until his INR is therapeutic. Disappointed for the delay in discharge, darn!!

I'm so tired lately, cleaning and getting the house ready at night for Bob's return, cooking, spending all day at the hospital. This too will end and we will be home resting soon, I hope and pray. Last day of February - Wow what a month!!!

Another busy morning with doctors doing their rounds, talking about maybe sucking out the blood clot so he can get off the blood thinners, but will call in another specialist to get an opinion. Went to the gym with PT and did ten minutes on the NuStep machine. Returned to the room, and his gown and pants were all wet; he is leaking from his tube sites. The nurse gets him cleaned up, changes the dressings, takes vitals etc.

The specialist comes by to see Bob's arm and also talked about maybe sucking out the clot; the doctors will confer and come up with a decision or plan.

We talked to the couple from the meeting; he got on the list today. We are so happy for him, now "all" he has to do is wait.

Cardiac rehab, another nap; he sleeps a lot because his red blood count is low and he is taking iron to help build it back up. Until it comes within normal range he will be tired; it will just take time.

March 3rd, 11 days post transplant and Bob is not feeling well today. His stomach is upset, probably from all the new meds, so we rest. During the doctors' rounds this morning, the pacemaker wires come out and they said that everything's looking good.

He is very grumpy today; I know he doesn't feel well, but I have been through a lot with him. You would think he could control how he reacts to me. Went for a short walk, and he either complains about exercise, walking, his mask, he's tired, his arm aches; it seems to always be something. I guess he is tired of hospitals, and I can't blame him. He snapped at me when I mentioned walking or getting dressed, so I have decided that I'm not going to ask him if he wants to do something. He needs to start making those decisions. If he doesn't say anything, then I'm not going to either. I have been in charge for a long time and I AM TIRED!!! He is getting well and needs to start making these decisions.

I decided it was time to take a break, so I went shopping for Bob's birthday and did a little therapy shopping as well; got a couple of nice tops. It made me feel a little better, as shopping usually does.

While I was gone, Bob had a two-hour nap. He wanted to go for a walk, so we did. Watched a video with information on what to do and know after you leave the hospital.

On my way to the cafeteria I stopped by the room of the man who just got on the list, to see if he needed or wanted anything. His wife had to go home for a few days, and his brother had not arrived yet, so I told him that I can stop and get him whatever he needs, just let me know. He said he was fine.

The next day Bob worked out in the gym. He said they changed his diet again because his potassium is too high, so now we also have to watch how much potassium is in the food he eats. High potassium can cause heart arrhythmia, so until he gets back to normal range, no tomato based sauces or other food high in potassium - just one more thing to keep track of.

It was a swinging door today with OT, PT, doctors,

nurses, and the nutritionist. Our social worker, who was on vacation when Bob got his heart, came by and was so happy for us, and it was good to see her as well. While we were talking with her, the diabetic educator wanted to come in, and I said NO, that we have someone else in here. She wasn't happy with us, but too bad, we had company. So after all this commotion, the nurse put a sign on the door that said to see the nurse before entering, so when we don't what to be disturbed or we are napping, we can let her know and put up the sign. It sure helped after that.

Bob didn't eat much for lunch; he just wasn't feeling well. He managed a walk outside and back, then a little dinner, and I left for home to fix dinner and lunch for tomorrow.

March 5th, HAPPY 60th BIRTHDAY Bob

Usual morning, but on my way to the hospital I bought birthday balloons, and when I arrived he was waiting to have a BM; the nurse gave him something to help and finally was able to have his BM and this made him feel a little better. Nurse was checking his blood sugar and he needs a little insulin. One of his anti-rejection meds can cause him to be diabetic, which we hope will not last too long. Some patients experience being a diabetic after transplant and others do not.

We had a nice lunch. Another blood draw and more meds to increase his heart rate. His Prograf was held back this morning, but then the nurse brought it at 2:00 p.m. with stat orders from the doctor. With his potassium high he gets a sugar pill to help lower his potassium, then insulin to help with the sugar; it is a balancing act.

It was a quiet afternoon, with birthday wishes from the staff, balloons and magazines and phone calls from friends, and Judy stopped by with birthday greetings as well.

Cardiac Rehab took Bob for a walk to ICU to see his nurses and doctors; they are so happy to see him doing well. We had a nice dinner I brought from home for this birthday, a little dessert, and then I left to go home.

As I left, I began to cry. I just don't know how much more I can do, with food restrictions, and watching Bob with his new heart - I would think he would be happier. We thought that after his transplant, life would be easier, but it is not. We are profoundly grateful for his new heart, and we just have to get through this little bump of managing meds, insulin, new diet restrictions, etc.

Next day was a beautiful morning for a walk, and I took advantage to clear my head and get ready for another day at the hospital. The nurse called me at 9:00 and said they are taking Bob for his biopsy, and the endocrinologist will be coming at 3:00 p.m. to go over taking insulin at home.

Well, this threw me over the edge; I had a major meltdown. Now we have this to deal with, besides high potassium, new heart meds, blood clots, kidneys not up to par... it is just a bit overwhelming this morning. So much for my nice "clear my head" walk.

When I arrived, a TP Coordinator was talking to Bob and said that these things are normal. They are working on adjusting his meds to help fix some of the issues that we are concerned about. It made us feel a little better, but still a lot to handle. His back and neck are hurting but he can't move for a while yet after his biopsy. Pain medication helps but also puts him to sleep until lunchtime, when he can move again.

We rested today. The appointment with the Endocrinologist, which went well, educated us on how to take and read his blood sugar levels and how much insulin to give, so when we go home we will know what to do.

The following couple of days Bob is looking and feeling better. He will be having monthly breathing treatments to take the place of his anti-bacterial medication called Bactrim. Bactrim can cause decreased kidney function and high potassium. The treatment will serve the same purpose without the side effects.

Results from his biopsy for rejection came back negative, potassium levels are coming down, and kidney function looks better today. Doctors said all this is attributed to getting a blood infusion yesterday; this is good news today. Also his bedsores are improving and his right arm where the blood clot is looks better as well. It's Friday and we have seen improvements, which makes me feel better; maybe I can get a good sleep tonight. It felt kind of strange, as today was also the first day in 132 days that I did not pack an overnight bag. News came that we may be going home on Monday, YEA!!

The weekend was busy with friends from Tucson visiting, getting ready to go home on Monday, also friends from Surprise stopped by on their way home from New Mexico. Just waiting around for Monday to come to see if we can go home.

The patient from California waiting for a heart got

word that there may be a heart for him, and he was taken to surgery on Saturday afternoon. His wife had decided to go home to California to take care of business, while his brother came to be with him. Wouldn't you know, she was only gone a day and he got the call they had a heart for him. We were all so happy for him, but he didn't tell his wife until later, when he knew for sure he was heading in to surgery. By the time she arrived back in Arizona, he was out of surgery and doing well. We came to know them over the next couple of months, as they had to stay close to the hospital for three months and we would see them from time to time in the cafeteria and attending appointments. Such a nice couple; we made new friends, a happy time.

I left a little early on Saturday and Sunday to get ready for Bob's homecoming on Monday, made soup, grocery shopped etc.

Chapter 6

Going Home

March 11th, 2013. Arriving earlier than usual on Monday morning, so excited that we are finally going home after 136 days since October of 2012, and 19 days post transplant.

Bob had a restless night with BM's and peeing. He was given meds to help him and it finally kicked in, so he slept most of the morning while we waited for the discharge paperwork. I finished packing his things; we met with the TP Coordinator and went over his medication, and received more education on taking care of himself after transplant.

We asked about when to shower and he can do that at any time, just watch the sites from his driveline and drainage tubes for infection. It's 4:00 p.m. and we are meeting with our nurse to go over the discharge instructions, filled the rest of his meds at the pharmacy, and then we are released.

Picked up PF Chang's takeout for dinner, went over the medication list, and did our insulin check before dinner.

It was all a little confusing but we managed; just so good to be home relaxing and getting to bed early. Something new for me to be home so early, and not up late cleaning, cooking, doing laundry etc. What a nice evening.

Our first morning to sleep in and not have to get ready to go to the hospital in 137 days, and the phone rings at 7:00 a.m. - it was the specialty pharmacy. I was not happy! They said they don't call before 9:00 a.m., and I replied, "Well, it's 7:00 a.m. here!"

We finished our business and it was time to get Bob up to check his blood, take his insulin, and eat breakfast, all so he can take his meds at 8:00 a.m. as scheduled. We had a little disagreement over his meds, but we are tired and nervous that we get it right. He is asking me questions about his meds, what pills do what etc., and we finally got it all figured out.

Later in the day we went to pick up the remainder of the vitamins that they want him to take. So we got out for a little walk at the store, then napped, had a nice dinner at home, watching TV, all is well.

It's day 2 at home. We are getting a routine - I wake Bob for his morning pill, we sleep for another twenty minutes, we get up, check blood sugar, give insulin. I have to give him his shot, since he shakes so badly from one of his meds that he can't hold the needle still to inject his insulin. The shakes will subside in time.

At 8:00 a.m., he must take his anti-rejection meds with breakfast, check blood pressure, get weighed, check temperature; lots to do first thing in the morning, but we are getting it. Yesterday was a little disorganized - much better this morning. We have a nice relaxing day just being at home, walked around the cul-de-sac, and talked to a few neighbors. We need more of these days to get caught up from the last couple of years.

Over the next few weeks we continue with our weekly follow-up appointments and monthly biopsies; we have some good days and some bad. The bad days are when Bob is weak and doesn't feel like walking. I get frustrated wanting him to do more and he gets mad and says he is tired because he is anemic, but if he doesn't at least walk, how can he get stronger?

I noticed one day that he was losing some hair from the back of his head, the size of a silver dollar, where he had a bed sore, but also some patients can lose hair from the meds they are on as well. When I went to brush it, more hair came off, so I guess he may lose his hair. Oh well, it will grow back; this is minor compared to the other things we have to deal with.

Another bad day would consist of Bob not making it to the bathroom in time, and then we have a Code Brown and have to clean him up and his clothes as well. This can happen because of weak muscles. When someone tells you that they have lost muscle mass, it can and did mean for Bob all of his muscles, including his rectum. So you see, it is not an easy time. We carry extra underwear and cleaning wipes when we go out, in case he has an accident.

We were at Sam's Club shopping, and Bob had to go to the restroom. He just made it, and I waited outside of the restroom for twenty minutes; he was having trouble getting off the toilet. The handicap stall was in use, and the others are too low for Bob to get off. He worked up the nerve to ask the attendant for help getting up off the toilet.

When he came out of the restroom he looked frazzled, and told me what had happened, then began to cry saying, "I want to be well again." He was sobbing and I was hugging him, telling him it will all be okay. We checked out and went home.

There are many more of these types of incidents over the next few months, but we manage. Now when he can't get up he phones me, and I can either go in or send help in for him.

It makes me sad when we go to our appointments and I see other TP patients up walking and strong, while Bob is weak, anemic, losing muscle mass, having to take insulin, doesn't feel like eating, sleeps a lot, etc. Then again, I think others have not been through what we have, so I try and look at the bright side, that this too will take time.

Another incident was when I left him off at the grocery store front door. I looked into my review mirror and he was on the ground. He had to step up onto the curb, didn't make it and fell. An employee and a man passing by came over and helped him up. We were both shaken. An employee brought a riding cart to get him around the store since he was shaken up from the fall.

It is now April, two months after TP. You would think he would be getting stronger but he just seems so weak. How I keep going I do not know. I am so fed up with this situation and Bob not having energy. His new heart is working great, but he does not want to do anything. I just don't know, I am thinking is it worth it, do I want to give up, these things go through my mind.

Maybe he has sleep apnea again, so they check his oxygen levels at night and they did fall below the recommended levels, so back to the Bipap machine to sleep. Between this and rehab we pray he will start to have more energy.

I ask for help setting up his Bipap equipment, and he just sits there, or when I talk about a new water heater, he just sits there. I finally said, "If I have to make decisions by myself I may as well live by myself," and, "You had a heart surgery, you didn't have brain surgery." I am just so tired and frustrated.

Bob looks so sad these last few weeks since he has been home and losing muscle mass. His clothes are too big, but he doesn't care about his looks. He only wants to take a couple of showers a week, saying it's too much work. Doesn't shave but once or twice a week, when we have appointments. Not the rather fastidious Bob I know; just doesn't care and this is so sad.

TP Coordinator called one day, checking up on us to see how we are doing. When I told her, she was wondering if they should admit him. I said, "What can you do that I'm not already doing?" and she said, "Nothing really, just wanted to make sure you are okay at home." I told her that we are, but sometimes I do think maybe Bob should go back in, and give me a break. I get tired from frustration at the end of the day - he has no motivation or desire to help himself, WHY???

Seven weeks post transplant and we have an appointment that will give us time to talk to the staff about Bob's condition and what we can do. The nurses are asking questions and reinforcing Bob's activity and how important it is that he gets moving. Rehab will start soon, so this should help a lot - at least it will be *them* telling him to get moving and not me nagging on him.

Before we left, we talked with the Social Worker about how maybe Bob is depressed. Sleeping a lot is a first sign of depression, as is low energy. She suggested we see the psychiatrist and to give it a week or so and see what happens. After talking to everyone today maybe he will pick up the pace and try to be more active.

A week later, with his blood draw they are testing for CMV, a virus that can lay dormant. The donor had signs of it but Bob did not. A few adjustments are made to his meds, including one called Cellcept that can cause diarrhea.

Five nights now back on the Bipap machine, and he seems to be feeling a little better. His sleep apnea really took a toll on his attitude, behavior, eating; what a difference it made. He has lost 30 pounds in the last month. The diarrhea he has been having seems to be getting better as well. Since he feels better, I do too.

Going for another biopsy today, we are up early for the blood draw. Once they take Bob to the Cath Lab for his procedure, I leave to go do a little shopping and meet Judy for lunch. But I got a phone call and the procedure is off, due to his INR being high, so I go back and get Bob, then the three of us go for lunch. Sad, my day of fun and friends is off once again.

April 23rd, Tuesday. Starting Rehab, Bob likes the trainers and they like him, just a reorientation into the routine. He did well on all three machines for a total of sixteen minutes, a good day at Rehab. He said he feels better and has more energy. I told him that it's the endorphins kicking in; energy creates energy. We will continue with Rehab three days a week for twelve weeks.

Thursday, he is scheduled for another biopsy since

the last one his INR was too high. While he was in his procedure, I run a few errands and when I arrive back he is ready to go home. His blood work came back that his white blood count was low, so we are to stay away from the malls and busy places where he could catch something. We are hopeful that instead of doing a Biopsy through the groin to check for rejection, they will be able to do a test through the blood called an "Allomap," which can detect rejection.

I know I keep saying how tired I am of this ordeal, with Bob not helping himself, all the appointments, waiting around, driving, early mornings, rehab etc. I guess it wouldn't seem so trying if only I felt Bob would try more and make an effort; then I could see progress. He has been home six weeks, and nine weeks post TP. Our friend from California is doing so well, strong, walking; he just has more desire and determination than I see in Bob.

A few days later I had a major meltdown, upset again in sooo many ways. I thought life would be happy after TP. Well, it's not. He doesn't seem happy, doesn't do anything, just sleeps and asks for this and that. He still needs help getting off the couch; I just thought he would be further along. A month after his LVAD he wanted to go to ballgames, movies etc., and now nothing!!! I cried a lot today, I am sad for Bob and for us. I would love to get someone to come and stay with him for a few days so I can get a break and just recharge. I so need a break, or Bob to start acting like he is happy about his heart and starting a new life. He seems so sad, old and weak, no energy, no desire to do anything, GOD HELP US!!!

The next few weeks until Wednesday, May 22nd, much

of the same routine with Rehab, doctor appointments, Bob sleeping and really not doing much of anything. We had an early appointment for blood work at 7:30 a.m., chest x-ray, ECHO, went for lunch, back for our afternoon appointment at the clinic.

Doctors wanted a CT Scan, and we had to go to the other clinic for that, twenty-five minutes away, and then home in rush hour traffic. Just as we were getting home the TP coordinator called and they found pneumonia in his right lung and want him in the hospital. So we packed a few things and went back, where Bob was admitted at 7:15 p.m. I stayed until 8:45 and then back home, another forty-five minute drive. I put some things together for Bob and tried to sleep, but it was after 1:00 a.m., and I was still awake.

The next two weeks were spent in the hospital taking cultures from his lung to figure out what strain of pneumonia it was, and taking heavy doses of antibiotics. Infectious Disease asked many questions about his lungs, like any coughing, no, fever, no, basically how he was feeling, and Bob answered, just tired and no energy.

While in the hospital, the kidney doctor was in to do an assessment and also order an ultrasound for his bladder and kidneys, checking for CDIFF since he has been having more than usual diarrhea.

Endocrinology came to adjust his insulin and told him to check his sugars, but no insulin unless it goes above 180, and so far it has not. It would be one less thing to worry about doing.

Another ultra sound for his swollen arm to see how the blood clot is coming along. We find out that there is no clot; it is dissolved. Great news, maybe he can get off the blood thinners.

A couple of days after arriving we found out one of the cultures came back positive for Nocardia Pneumonia. It's a really nasty infection/bug that targets a lot of TP patients and people with a low immune system. It will be treated with heavy antibiotics, IV and pills for now. We will have to wait until next week for more information since it is a long weekend with Memorial Day on Monday.

The kidney doctor that was in said it could take a year or two to get over this infection, but we aren't getting excited until we talk to the Infections Disease (ID) Doctor. He will know more and can answer our questions, so for now it's wait and relax for today.

Home again, and I have been thinking what another sad day for us, with this infection setting Bob back. This is why he has not recovered from the heart surgery, having this infection lurking in his lungs. Now I feel bad that I have been so hard on Bob and his recovery.

If it does take a year or two to get rid of this, I have questions that need to be answered. Like, how long in the hospital, will he have a normal life, how will it affect his rehab and getting stronger? I went to bed and had a good cry; so much has happened. Still not asleep at midnight, so I got up and had a cup of tea. So worried!! I hope we can get more answers tomorrow. My stomach is in knots, just worrying about what will be next!!

Next day, the ID Doctor came in and said they are waiting to find out what strain of Nocardia it is, so that they can target it with the right meds, but until then we will stay the course we are on. It will take six months on heavy antibiotics, and then we will check the lung again to make sure it is gone. This is better news than we heard yesterday (that it could take two years.)

Psychiatrist was in to talk to Bob about his moods and activity level. She doesn't think he is going through anything unusual nor does she think he is depressed, but would like to adjust and change his mood medication.

We moved to a larger room with a table and chairs, two recliners, much more comfortable. Even though it is a holiday, Bob gets to the gym with PT, and has a good workout. So overall a pretty good day, and I am feeling more at ease as well.

Another day with another worry - one of the PA's was in and thought Bob looked a little odd. His mouth looked like it was droopy, so he did all the tests to see if maybe he had a stroke. He passed the tests with no problem; Bob was fine. That being said, the word got around and now they are going to do a CT Scan of his head to make sure he didn't have a stroke. Also a speech therapist was in doing tests for memory, numbers etc. He did not score well on one of the tests.

Bob is very chatty today, talking more that I have heard or seen in years; he said he feels good and he is happy for the first time since Transplant. He keeps on chatting most of the day keeping nurses, doctors, PA's etc. longer than needed; he just wants to talk. He is really very funny. I was talking to a social workers and she said, "Boy, he is sure talkative today." That's when I realized that they had changed one of his mood meds and he started the new one this morning. She said to keep an eye on him, and if his mood doesn't calm down, to let the nurse know.

The next day he was much calmer, it was just a reaction to the change of meds. Continuing on with the evaluation from what they thought may have been a stroke, Neurology was in and asked questions about seeing things, head trauma, sight, hearing, meningitis, asked him to walk and do a few other tasks. He had a CT Scan for his head, but no result by the time I left for the night.

My worry now is his brain. The PA indicated that the infection/pneumonia can go to the brain, and they want to make sure it has not. So this is why all the testing today. I am so worried that he is going to die from this infection. Needless to say I did not sleep well that night.

As I was leaving the house the next morning, Bob called and told me the scan came back NORMAL. We were so happy, I cried, what a relief.

We had thought we might be going home soon, but they changed his antibiotics, and want to watch him for a few more days for any reaction. Also he has some fluids they would like to get off him, and they can watch his kidney function and regulate his meds better if he stays. Makes sense, so we stay and wait.

Since they found the pneumonia and have been treating him, Bob is feeling so much better, with more energy. I think he is finally truly on his way to recovery.

A couple of days later we are ready to go home with an IV antibiotic. Home care doesn't arrive until 11:30 and then it was 12:30 p.m. before they left. I hope I remember what to do, since I will be changing his IV meds three times a day every eight hours for about a month or more. It's not a problem, as I used to change his other IV meds in the past.

Nice to be home; now we can get on track to recovery

and back to Rehab, getting Bob stronger and well again. He is doing so much better, helping a little more around the house, and not using walking poles for support as often. He has made such a change since we entered the hospital this last time until now. He is alive again. It's the best he has been since his TP in February, so good to finally see progress.

As June arrives, Bob is doing better each day. He is alive! A little slow on his reactions and thinking, he sometimes can't remember things and appointments, but that is why I am his Care Giver. It all takes time and patience, but who would have thought it would take this long? Some patients bounce right back. They are driving, walking, and are strong right away, living life within weeks, but Bob has had a rough road. Maybe because of all his previous surgeries it takes longer for the body to recover, so we are told.

As for me, I am doing better too, less stress when I can see improvement in his eating, walking and his demeanor. He has a better outlook on life. It is what I expected him to be after TP. It has taken longer, but at least it is happening. I am still jumpy and want to cater to him, but I am letting him do more for himself, which is good. It will help him get stronger and build confidence. I think we can see the light.

The rest of the month we continue Rehab and med changes. He is taken off his IV antibiotic and now is just on oral antibiotics for the next six months. The ID doctor said he should be just fine and that the infection has not spread. It was a good thing they caught it early, because it could have spread to other parts of the body, arms, brain, organs, and this could have been deadly.

June 23rd was a day that Bob was tired and seemed to be going to the bathroom more than usual. Then around 5:30 p.m. he complained about a pain in his right side, but ate dinner. The pain got worse, so he took an OXY, but that didn't seem to help, so we called the TP coordinator and went to the emergency room.

He was in such pain that he was shaking. It took a long time to get him medication for the pain but when he finally got it he settled down. A CT scan to see if it is kidney stones, and at 11:00 p.m. the results showed that it was indeed a stone, so more medication to help with pain and an anti-inflammatory. Discharged and home by 12:30 a.m., tired - yet another bump in the road.

I have been thinking today about friends and family. Some friends from Tucson came to visit in February right after Bob's transplant and said they would keep in touch and want to get together more. Well, that was in February and we haven't heard from them since. Also a cousin of mine - I haven't heard from her since before Christmas. I thought we were close, but not an email or phone call all these months. Another second cousin spends the winters in Phoenix area, has a home twenty minutes away and no word from them. So it is sad to think that there are some friends and family that just are too busy to care. At least, that's how it feels. It's okay; we know who our true friends are. They call, email, and chat online. As Bob says, "When you get sick you find out who your real friends are." It's true, but a little sad as well.

We are starting to do more, go to baseball games, movies etc. In between doctor appointments and rehab, we seem to keep busy.

One day while waiting for an appointment, as we watch people come and go, we realize although we have been through so much, and it has taken Bob a long time to recover, that we are lucky. There are so many people in wheelchairs that are there for the rest of their lives, people who have lost their sight, cancer patients, and people who need other organs, and who knows what else. They look really sick, so we consider ourselves blessed that Bob is on his way to living a full life.

We shop for new clothes; Bob needs a suit for his niece's wedding in August. He has lost so much weight that his clothes are all too big.

Sadly, Bob's Mom passed away on July 21st. Luckily the doctors said it is fine to travel, but to take precautions from germs, wear his mask, wipe down the plane seats and trays with wipes etc. We make the trip back to Michigan for the funeral service, leaving on July 25th and returning on the 28th. This is our first trip in years and I'm a little nervous. Bob says he is fine, and the trip went really well. Although it was for a sad occasion, it was nice to spend time with his side of the family.

August 2013 is a busy time. Wow, where has the time gone? It seems like just yesterday that Bob was getting his heart and I was helping him do everything, shower, dress, walking with walking sticks to help his balance, and now he is doing so much on his own. I remember when I thought this would never end and there was no light at the end of the tunnel, but there is, and it's so good to see him fixing his own meals, showering on his own, etc.

He has finished Rehab, so we continue to go to our own gym to work on his strength training. We need to work on his driving, so he can feel more independent and get out and do things on his own. We begin his driving with me in the car, going to or returning from the grocery store. Then he went out on a few short drives by himself. This all took place over a few weeks, but eventually he was feeling comfortable again behind the wheel.

He has been talking about getting back to golf, and all the things he hasn't been able to do. All this is good to see and hear.

August 11th, Bob wakes at 7:15 a.m. with kidney stones again. We head over to the Emergency Room, where he received pain medication, since what we have at home didn't seem to help, also another CT Scan. Neurology checked in and they want to keep him overnight for pain management and to watch his kidney function, since his Creatin was 2.9 this morning, and that is high. We also wait to talk to the heart team, to see if they could go in and break up and drain out the stones. He has one that is 3 mm, ready to go into the bladder to be passed, and a couple more floating around.

It is possible they may do a procedure tomorrow, to go in and get the stones. My question is, will they still do it with him being on Coumadin (blood thinner)? The PA will check.

An Ultrasound is scheduled for his right arm to see if the blood clots are still there; that is why he is on Coumadin. If the clots are gone, he may be able to stop taking it. I also mentioned to the nurse that he was taking a large amount of calcium after TP, and then he started to have these stones. He didn't have this problem before - just something to think about.

Monday the 12ᵗʰ, he went for his procedure, but they couldn't go in and get the stones since his INR was too high. They did place a stent to help drain the kidneys. His urine was dark and cloudy, possible infection, so it was decided to wait until the kidneys settle down. The Creatin is better to get the stones, or maybe the stones will pass on their own.

A couple more days in the hospital. Since we were there, we went to the Support group meeting and our friends from California were there. So good to see them and see that he is doing well since his TP.

Bob's labs looked better and we were discharged on Wednesday afternoon.

Tuesday, August 20, 2013. Today is a big milestone; six months post TP, and a big appointment day, where he had a great check-up. Doctors informed us he could drive, golf, and start living life. He is doing well and now we can get ready for our trip to Philadelphia for his niece's wedding.

Finished packing, cleaning house and to bed by 9:00 p.m, as we have a driver picking us up at 4:15 a.m. for the airport. A smooth flight, with breakfast and a couple of Bloody Mary's (for me, not Bob). After a long day of travel we arrived in Reading, Pennsylvania in time for dinner.

Friday we attended the Arizona Diamondbacks vs Philadelphia Phillies baseball game in Philadelphia, a beautiful evening for an outside game, after spending a hot summer in Arizona.

Saturday was the wedding at an old mansion in Reading, Pennsylvania. A beautiful wedding, outdoors, with bagpipes playing, Bob's brother dressed in his Navy uniform walking his daughter to the altar; it was a beautiful event.

The next day we drove to Warminster, Pennsylvania, where his brother lives and we stayed there for the rest of our visit. Taking in the sites of Philly - Independence Square, Liberty Bell, the Mint, Constitution Hall, riding the train downtown a couple of times, eating cheese steak sandwiches, etc. Another day we drove to the Jersey shore. Although it was very hot at the beach, we did a little tourist shopping and called it a day. Truly a fun week and Bob did amazingly well. I haven't seen him like this in years, really can't remember when, maybe fifteen years, energy, walking, enjoying life, such joy.

Arriving home on Friday, August 30th after a fun week, we had a few days to relax and then get ready for another trip. This time we drove to San Diego, California, for Bob's SME mid-year meeting Sept. 7-10th. It was such fun, and for Bob's friends who had been worrying about him all these months, to see him doing so well. He attended his meetings; we ate out, walked around the Gaslight district, and had a nice few days.

We arrived home on Sunday afternoon, had a light dinner, and suddenly Bob's pain started again. Oh no, not this again. He took a couple of painkillers, but that didn't help, so here we go again off to the Emergency Room, after a five hour drive, another 45 minutes...I am so tired! We were in the ER until 1:15 a.m., doing the usual labs, urine tests, CT Scan. Nothing showed up and then no more pain, so we were released to go home, tired and discouraged.

During the past couple of weeks, Bob has been talking to the HR department at work. Yes, he wants to go back to work, and the doctors do release him to do so after filling out paperwork, and asking questions such as what kind of job, are there chemicals, any hard labor, hours, etc.

He was released and able to go back to work as of October 1, 2013, after only seven months post TP, truly amazing. He is ready to go back. He is tired of being around the house, and wants to get on with life. Let's hope nothing happens to prevent this. We inform the company and we are told to hold on, that a position is coming available that they are working on.

A busy weekend of going to a baseball game on Saturday, followed by a Cardinals (football) game on Sunday, then a couple of days to relax before we drive back to California for my girlfriend Candy's son's wedding.

Candy and her husband Gonzalo arrive from Santiago, Chile, on Monday and we will meet up with them on Thursday. The bridal shower is Saturday, and the wedding on Sunday. We did a lot of walking, meeting up with friends we hadn't seen in a long time, a fun few days. Stayed for a couple of extra days, and drove home on Tuesday September 24th.

Chapter 7

Back To Work

By the 26ᵗʰ of September a job offer came from the company. He accepted, although the job is in Safford, Arizona, which is three hours away. The company will move us. We began a new journey in our lives; moving is such a big job. They say it is the hardest thing next to death and divorce. (I think a heart transplant should rank right up there too, haha.) This is move number fourteen for us, so you could say we are pros.

The weekend of October 12ᵗʰ, we move Bob into temporary housing, and I begin a home search. We were lucky to find one fast. Also, our home in Sun City West sold within a week. So off we go with moving. Busy couple months, but we get the homes closed and move into our home in Safford end of November.

Life is going along smoothly with work and going back and forth for follow-up appointments. Since we are not yet one year out from post TP, there are still a lot of appointments. Along about mid December, Bob's right leg seems to be getting bigger and retaining fluid; we are told to take Lasik, which will help with fluid retention.

At our next appointment the doctor looks at his leg and is confused, because his left leg is normal. He orders an ultrasound for his leg to make sure it is not a blood clot. None found, so good news. We then go back to the clinic and see another doctor. He also is confused and he calls in a Vascular doctor who he wants to do a CT Scan. He suspects that he may have an obstruction further up his groin.

Admitted into the hospital again. The next day Bob has his CT Scan and they find no blood clots and no obstructions. The only thing they can figure out is that perhaps scar tissue around the incision from having so many biopsies for his right heart cath has blocked a vein, and the fluids are not returning into his body, a condition called Lumphademia. Instruction is to elevate the leg and wear a support stocking to help with circulation. Also the doctor has written a prescription for a leg pump, which we will have to order.

After a month we finally find a compression pump and have it delivered. Bob must wear compression stockings daily and use the compression pump in the evenings for two hours. We are told there is nothing that can be done for Lumphademia, and he will have to live with his right leg being twice the size of his left. Bob has such a great attitude, he said, "I'm not going to let this stop me from doing what I want to do. I have been through so much I can live with this. I'm alive and working, that's all that matters."

We have a wonderful Christmas at home. Since the

last two Christmases were spent in the hospital, we are just happy to be home.

A quick business trip to Salt Lake City, and we stayed a few extra days to see his sons and their families. It was a good thing for the kids to see their Dad after all he had been through.

Epilogue

One Year and Beyond Post Transplant

February arrives and we are scheduled for his one-year follow up, lots of routine testing is being done - ECHO, chest X-ray, blood work, six-minute walk etc. He passed with flying colors, his Ejection Fraction is great, and all his labs were in line. He is doing superb, and they said, "Go home, enjoy life, and we will see you in a year unless you have any concerns or problems." Wow, what a terrific day, and then again, after being under their watchful eyes for so many years, it is kind of scary at the same time to be out on our own.

We return home, and begin living again; life is good. We not only see light at the end of the tunnel - we are through it. God is good.

We haven't started to golf yet, since the weather was too cold in the winter and then too hot in the summer, but we are looking forward to beginning again in spring and autumn.

Bob continues working, and traveling for work. We took a vacation to the Upper Peninsula of Michigan for a week in June of 2014, and Bob and his son Derek attended the Michigan/Notre Dame game at Notre Dame in September 2014. 4 Years Post Transplant we are still making plans for more travel, vacations, possible retirement etc.

Death Was Not An Option

By: Robert (Bob) Washnock

"Lately it occurs to me, what a long, strange trip it's been." No truer words were ever spoken about my life for the past sixteen years. Thanks to the Grateful Dead for this lyric.

When I reflect back on my childhood and friends, death never entered our minds; it was all about playing sports, climbing trees, visiting with friends, running and laughing. We played football on our neighborhood streets, only to be interrupted by the occasional car. We would shout "car!" clear the street, and once the car passed by, "game on!" and we played on. We played pond hockey on any sheet of ice we could find, never wore a helmet or face mask, never got cut or hit with a stick or puck, never thought we could be injured.

I fell from a tree once, only to unconsciously reach out and grab a branch that prevented me from hitting the ground. Scary, but I didn't think about the consequences and kept climbing trees. I dislocated my ankle playing softball, sliding into second base. My foot turned under the bag; I heard a pop, looked down and saw my right foot extending outward at a forty-five degree angle from my leg. Then the pain came; it felt like my ankle was in a vise and the vise kept getting tighter and tighter. My only concern was whether I would be able to play softball again that summer. Never a conscious thought about my own mortality.

All of that changed when I turned forty-four, and I was walking up just a slight incline at work and experienced shortness of breath. It was difficult to catch my breath and I had to stop and continually take deep breaths. I thought, "What is up with this?" I immediately made an appointment to see my doctor; I was scared, never having experienced something like this before. I was always healthy growing up, with occasional pains and strains from playing sports, and a yearly bout with strep throat during my pre-teens.

When I first visited my general practitioner following the shortness of breath incident, he said he could hear PVC's when listening to my heart. I asked, "What are those?" "Pre-ventricular contractions," he said. "Is that serious?" I asked, and he replied, "They can be." He referred me to a cardiologist to get a detailed diagnosis of my problem.

Once at the cardiology clinic, the doctor performed an echocardiogram (echo) on my heart. When the results were ready, he called me to come in and discuss. He informed me that I had dilated cardiomyopathy, a degenerative weakening of the heart muscle, and my left ventricle was enlarged. He went on to say that my ejection fraction (EF) was only 19% and normal EF is in the range of 50% to 70%. I said, "Okay Doc, what does it all mean?" He said, "With time the heart muscle will grow weaker, thereby decreasing blood flow through your body, and eventually you will need a heart transplant. Your EF is low and that's why you were feeling out of breath. We can control some of these symptoms now with medication."

I said to myself, "WOW, this can't be true, I've been healthy my entire life. Why am I facing these health issues at age forty-four? There must be some mistake." Naturally I could not accept this news and ultimately I was in denial. My doctor prescribed the appropriate medications and I took the pills on good faith.

My health seemed to stabilize over the next three years and in the interim I began to see a cardiologist. In 2000, my heart started to experience ventricular tachycardia (V-tach), an arrhythmia that could be fatal. My cardiologist insisted that I have an implantable cardio-defibrillator (ICD) installed in my chest so that my heart could be shocked out of any type of arrhythmia.

My first defibrillator was implanted in March of 2000. The first time it shocked me was after a round of golf. I was putting my golf glove back in the bag and all of a sudden it felt like something hit me in the back of the head. I was stunned for a minute thinking I had been hit by a golf ball, but finally realized the defibrillator had shocked me. I proceeded to go back into the clubhouse and really did not give the incident much thought.

The defibrillator shocked me out of bad arrhythmias about one hundred fifty times over the next eleven years. The shocks did not hurt, just scared the heck out of me, and it felt like a mule was kicking me in the chest.

Over this time period the defibrillator shocked me so hard that it knocked me off stools, I fainted twice due to the extremely fast heart rate, and I developed PTSD (post-traumatic stress disorder). My life with a defibrillator was a living hell. Every time I felt my heart flutter I braced myself for a shock. Sometimes it never came, other times it hit me and I would be frightened of more shocks for several days. If the defibrillator shocked me more than two times in an hour it meant a trip to the hospital emergency room and an IV medicine to calm the heart rhythm. Several of these hospital trips occurred in this time period. Most were overnight stays and some resulted in several days in the hospital.

My heart continued to get weaker over the years and I started to get short of breath. My blood flow was slowing down due to the weakened heart muscle; it could not send enough blood to the lungs to get oxygenated. In August of 2011, I went to see my EP cardiologist. He performed some tests and informed me that my EF was now only 8%. He said that he could do nothing more for me, and it was time to investigate the possibility of a heart transplant.

Following his advice, I contacted the Mayo Clinic in Phoenix, Arizona. The heart doctors there had evaluated me before, so they were familiar with my condition. I scheduled an office visit in October 2011, and after the doctor examined me he informed me that I should go home for the weekend and be prepared to be hospitalized on the following Monday. He said that my heart condition was serious and that I needed to have pre-transplant testing for a transplant. This began my two-year journey of hospital stays, medical testing, surgeries, and recovery periods.

I realized that my battle for life was just beginning

and I needed to prepare myself for what was to come. I was scared of the unknown and what lay ahead for me. I thought to myself, "I must be brave, commit to getting well, and put my life in the hands of my doctors." I told myself over and over, "I can beat this, I can get well and strong again, and I can overcome any of the medical procedures and surgeries that are necessary. I'm going to be tough, strong, resilient, tenacious, and fight all the way. After all, I still have a lot to live for." I wanted to see my grandkids grow up, spend more time with my beautiful wife, desired to continue working in my profession, and I still had a lot to learn and offer in life.

My trials and tribulations with heart disease, the LVAD implant, and ultimately the heart transplant and subsequent complications are well documented in this book.

The objective of this book is to reach out to people who are facing crises in their life, whether it is serious health conditions, perceived insurmountable odds in life, terminal diseases, depression, or those who consider that life is no longer worth living.

What is paramount is hope; never give up hope, and know that there are friends, family, and colleagues that love you and care for you. You are not alone.

Jimmy Valvano, former head basketball coach at North Carolina State University and inspirational speaker, dying of terminal brain cancer said, "Don't give up, don't ever give up." He fought the cancer with all the strength he had. In Mr. Valvano's acceptance speech for the 1993 inaugural ESPY Awards – The Arthur Ashe Courage Award, he said, "Cancer can take away all of my physical abilities; it cannot touch my mind, it cannot touch my heart and it cannot touch my soul and those three things are gonna carry on forever."

Before he passed, Jimmy formed the V Foundation and to date they have donated over $170 million to cancer research. Jimmy V, as he was affectionately known, always felt he would beat the cancer.

Another inspiration to me was Stuart Scott, an accomplished sports broadcaster for ESPN, who contracted a rare form of appendiceal cancer. After his "chemo" treatments he would go to the gym and workout for hours. Stuart knew he had to keep his strength to fight the disease. He was defiant of the disease, saying many times, "FU to cancer." During his acceptance speech for the 2014 Jimmy V Perseverance ESPY Award, Stuart said, "You beat cancer by how you live, why you live, and the manner in which you live." The same can be said for any disease or situation that we confront in life. During that same speech Stuart went on to say, "So live, live, fight like hell, and when you get too tired to fight, lay down and rest and let someone else fight for you." Stewart also admitted that he could not do this "don't give up thing" by himself. He stated that he had thousands of people on Twitter, on the streets, at work and his family who encourage and add to his fight. Mr. Scott also stated, "This whole fight thing, this journey thing, is not a solo journey, it requires support."

My lessons learned during this difficult period in my life are as follows:

1. Change your thinking, be positive, and fight. The power of positive thinking will work for you in unbelievable ways.

2. Commit to getting well and regaining health.
3. Set goals for yourself in your recovery and what you want to accomplish when you get well.
4. Know and trust that modern medicine and science can save your life.
5. Put your life in the hands of your doctors and nurses.
6. Ask questions about recommended procedures and medicines. Why are we doing this and what information or benefit do we hope to gain? Seek to understand all that is proposed and what your doctors will perform.
7. Your caregiver is the most important person in your life. My wife, Pam, showed me what unconditional love was all about. When I was too tired to fight she fought for me, she kicked me in the butt when I most needed it and above all else she was a huge support for me. She was there every day for me - my strength, my inspiration, my support, and my love. She endured more than I did as the patient because she was there for all of it. I was sedated many times and short-term memory loss is an after effect of these drugs.
8. You are not alone in your fight; your doctors, nurses, friends, colleagues and family will all fight for and with you.
9. Be courageous in your fight. Courage is not without fear; courage is acting, fighting in the face of those fears.

I am convinced that had I not changed my attitude, used the power of positive thinking, set goals for myself, developed a strong will to live and followed my doctors' recommendations, I would not be here today. I was very fortunate to have received the best medical care possible at the Mayo Clinic near Phoenix, Arizona. The doctors, nurses, and staff who cared for and supported me are also responsible for saving my life.

Our goal is to inspire those who are patients, caregivers, or anyone who may be facing life-altering situations that there is hope; there are many good reasons to fight the fight and to live your life. It is our sincere hope that this book can help and give you solace on your journey.

"Don't give up, don't ever give up."

THE END

Mayo Hospital Staff

Here are just a few of the hospital staff
who had a hand in our journey.

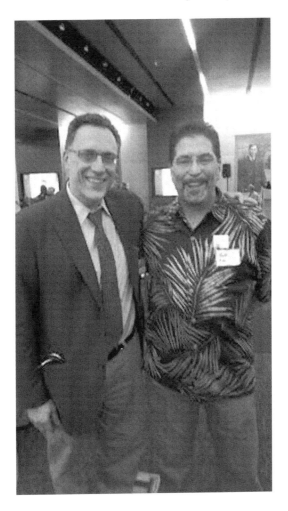

Dr. Pajaro, one of the Thoracic Surgeons
who Transplanted Bob's Heart

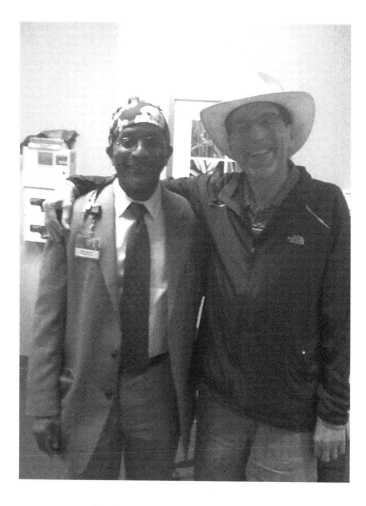

Dr. Scott, one of the Cardiologists

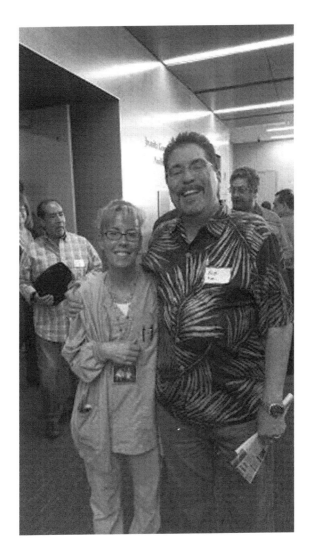

Linda, one of the LVAD Coordinators

Medications

After Transplant Medications: There are many types of anti-rejection drugs; I have listed the ones Bob was on and some he will be on for the rest of his life.

Immunosuppressant Medications: Suppress or decrease your immune system to prevent rejection of the donor heart.

Prednisone is a member of the class of medications called corticosteroids or steroids and comes in tablet or IV form. It occurs naturally in the body and is produced by the adrenal glands (glands that produce a range of hormones). Important in preventing the body from rejecting the transplanted heart.

Mycophenolate mofetil (Cellcept) is a drug that reduces the white blood cell count.

Tacrolimus (Prograf) works to prevent and treat rejection by suppressing the activity of the immune cells.

Sirolimus (Rapamune) is an immunosuppressant.

Fluconazole Antifungal medication, used to treat and prevent fungal infections.

Valcyte Antiviral medication, used to treat viral infections.

Bactrim Antibacterial medication, used to treat or prevent infections caused by bacteria.

Simvastatin Lowers high cholesterol and triglycerides. Studies have found statin therapy initiated early in the postoperative period plays an important role for better survival and lower incidence of transplant vasculopathy (a disorder of blood vessels).

Current Transplant Medications for life:

Tacrolimus (Prograf)
Sirolimus (Rapamune)
Simvastatin,
Aspirin 81mg

Other Terminology:

ECHO (Echocardiogram): Test in which pulses of sound (ultrasound) are sent into the body and the ECHOs returning from the surfaces of the heart produce images that are recorded.

Heart Catheterization (Cath): Procedure in which a catheter is inserted into the heart to assess pressures and the condition of coronary arteries, valves, and heart muscle.

Endomyocardial Biopsy: A test to tell if rejection is occurring. The procedure involves taking a small piece of tissue from the heart, usually from the right ventricle, through a vein in the neck or leg.

Rejection: A complication of transplantation in which the immune system recognizes the donor heart as "foreign" and tries to destroy it.

Ventilator: A machine that assists a person's breathing (also known as a respirator)

Additional Information:

What are the OPTN and UNOS?

The Organ Procurement and Transplantation Network (OPTN) links all of the professionals involved in the nation's organ donation and transplantation system. The OPTN also strives to make more organs available and increases patient access for transplants.

The *United Network of Organ Sharing (UNOS)*: A non-profit organization that operates under a contract from the federal government, licensed by the U.S. Government to provide matching of organ donors and recipients. www. unos.org

The OPTN and UNOS continuously review new advances in research and use this information to improve organ transplant policies to best serve patients needing transplants. All transplant programs and organ procurement organizations are members of the OPTN and agree to follow its policies.

Made in the USA
Middletown, DE
07 May 2021

39165320R00109